D0852105

MECHANICAL LOW BACK PAIN

Perspectives in Functional Anatomy

MECHANICAL
LOW BACK PAIN

Perspectives in Functional Anatomy

JAMES A. PORTERFIELD, P.T., M.A., A.T.C.

President, Rehabilitation and Health Center, Crystal Clinic
  Akron, Ohio
Assistant Professor, Cleveland State University
  Cleveland, Ohio

CARL DeROSA, P.T., M.S.

Associate Professor and Chairman, Physical Therapy Program
Northern Arizona University
  Flagstaff, Arizona

1991
W.B. SAUNDERS COMPANY
Harcourt Brace Jovanovich, Inc.

PHILADELPHIA, LONDON, TORONTO, MONTREAL, SYDNEY, TOKYO

LIBRARY
ARAPAHOE COMMUNITY COLLEGE
2500 WEST COLLEGE DRIVE
P. O. BOX
LITTLETON, CO 80160-9002

W. B. SAUNDERS COMPANY
Harcourt Brace Jovanovich, Inc.

The Curtis Center
Independence Square West
Philadelphia, PA 19106

Library of Congress Cataloging-in-Publication Data

Porterfield, James A.

   Mechanical low back pain / by James A. Porterfield, Carl DeRosa.
      p.   cm.

   ISBN 0-7216-7297-3

   1. Backache—Pathophysiology.   2. Backache—Patients—
Rehabilitation.   I. DeRosa, Carl.   II. Title.   [DNLM: 1. Backache.
2. Biomechanics.   3. Lumbosacral region—physiology.
WE 755 P849m]
RD771.B217P67   1991   617.5′64—dc20
DNLM/DLC
90-8465

Sponsoring Editor: Margaret Biblis
Developmental Editor: Leslie E. Hoeltzel
Manuscript Editor: Barbara Hodgson
Designer: Lorraine B. Kilmer
Illustration Coordinator: Matthew Andrews
Production Manager: Frank Polizzano
Indexer: Susan Thomas

MECHANICAL LOW BACK PAIN   ISBN   0-7216-7297-3

Copyright © 1991 by W. B. Saunders Company.

All rights reserved. No part of this publication may be reproduced or transmitted in any form or by any means, electronic or mechanical, including photocopy, recording, or any information storage and retrieval system, without permission in writing from the publisher.

Printed in the United States of America.

Last digit is the print number: 9   8   7   6   5   4   3   2   1

With love to Marlene and Bonnie,
whose understanding and encouragement
provide us great personal strength and direction.

JAN 1 1992

ACKNOWLEDGMENTS

An undertaking of this sort demands that many individuals be given due recognition. Our early teachers in manual therapy, including Stanley Paris and Freddy Kaltenborn, provided us with an excellent foundation for further study.

Our fellow clinicians and faculty members with whom we work have also been sounding boards for MECHANICAL LOW BACK PAIN, especially Vince Secker, John McCulloch, Phil Sauer, Dave Roessler, and Tom McPoil.

We are also indebted to our students. They have continually provided us with the stimulus to continue learning and have challenged us in a way that has forced us to pursue more answers.

Last, we would like to acknowledge the help of our editors with manuscript preparation, and the work of Tina Cauller. Ms. Cauller's fine artwork and the editorial staff have allowed us to reach the goals we personally set out to attain in writing MECHANICAL LOW BACK PAIN.

PREFACE

Over the past few years there has been increasing recognition of the magnitude of low back pain problems. Interestingly, during the same time period that significant advances in technology and methods of intervention have surfaced, the problem itself has continued to proliferate, resulting in increasing societal costs.

Coincident with technological advances has been a dramatic increase in the understanding of the anatomy, biomechanics, and physiology of the low back. This new knowledge has in turn caused us to reformulate some of the evaluation and treatment ideas traditionally taught in the past. In recognition of this new knowledge, models of evaluation and treatment have gone through a maturational process.

In *MECHANICAL LOW BACK PAIN*, we have attempted to detail the functional anatomy of the low back. From such a foundation, a method of evaluation and treatment has been developed. We have attempted to interrelate the mechanical bases of function and dysfunction to evaluation and treatment. Perhaps more important, our textbook emphasizes the new direction of management: recognizing the important distinction between low back pain and low back disability.

No matter how sophisticated the technological advances, we believe that the ultimate goal of treatment will always be directed toward restoring function. As our understanding of the physical characteristics of low back tissues increases, we become more adept at keeping people active without compromising the tissues of the spine and at teaching the patient how to stress the spine within its physiological limits. Clinical experience and the literature support an active, rather than passive, approach toward rehabilitation. Our goal is to assist the reader of *MECHANICAL LOW BACK PAIN* in correlating current knowledge with a logical program of active management.

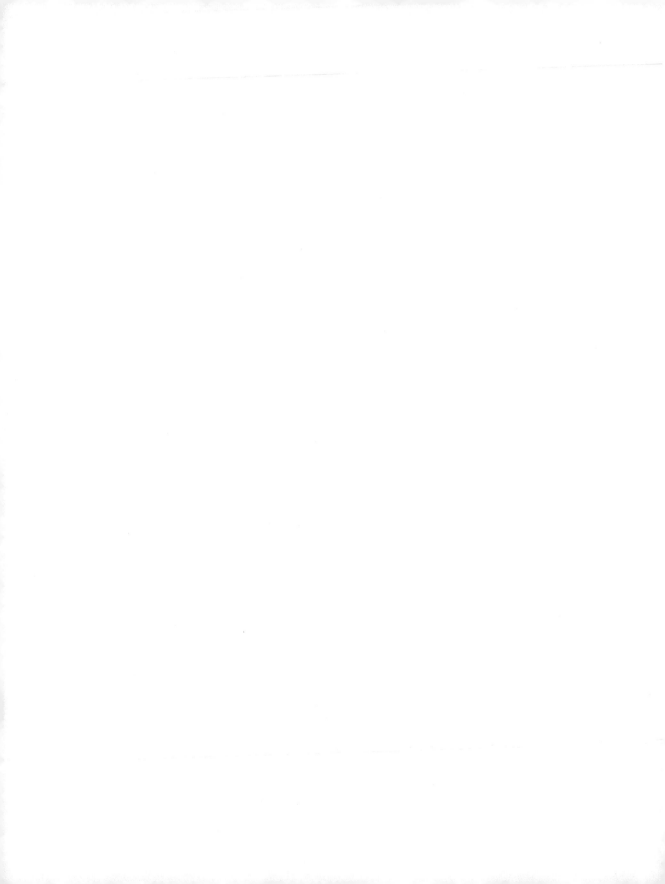

CONTENTS

1

PRINCIPLES OF MECHANICAL LOW BACK DISORDERS

THE LOW BACK DILEMMA

The magnitude of the low back disability problem has been noted in various epidemiological studies.[3,7,34,44,50] Disorders of the low back are currently the leading cause of disability in people under age 45.[37] Of the $27 billion spent on *all* musculoskeletal trauma, $16 billion is spent in the management of low back pain, with more than half of this latter amount spent on surgical treatment.[33,37]

Because of such staggering statistics, novel evaluation and treatment methods for low back disorders have continually been sought. Attempts to manage the problem have led to research resulting in new knowledge in anatomy, biomechanics, exercise physiology, and neurosciences. This expanding knowledge base has in turn resulted in the modification of some practice habits, the discarding of others, and the addition of new and innovative forms of treatment.

Clinical practice has also been continually reshaped by the political, socioeconomic, and legal climate. The rising cost of care for mechanical low back disorders has forced a reexamination of the payment schedules by various third party payers. This change in reimbursement attitudes for services that are provided has mandated new directions for treatment. Additionally, some clinicians have become hesitant to be involved with the industrial low back injury for reasons other than a dwindling reimbursement dollar. This hesitancy can be attributed in part to the perceived low success rate in attempting to manage these patients, as well as to the concern of being drawn into disputes that have resulted in litigation.

One of the primary reasons for the escalation of the low back dilemma is the difficulty in separating the predicament of low back pain from low back disability. Low back pain is essentially a universal and self-limiting phenomenon; it is so common that it can be considered a normal occurrence.[56] By contrast, low back disability is a relatively recent Western epidemic.[56] That is to say, although low back pain has been recognized and accepted as a fairly common occurrence, low back disability, as a distinct entity, has surfaced only in modern times. As we begin to better understand the difference between the two, approaches to evaluation and treatment necessarily change. Low back pain and low back disability need to be separated because if all low back pain is treated as if it were a disability, then what was previously a mechanical disorder has the potential to become an "illness."

It is well recognized that treating the patient with mechanical low back pain with activity decreases the disability, whereas treating the patient with prolonged rest, analgesics, and minimal activity increases the disability.[22] Furthermore, it has been demonstrated that pain behavior is inversely proportional to the amount of exercise done.[24] As a result of this understanding, the approach to the treatment of low back disorders is changing. Management of the problem has shifted from passive therapeutic interventions to more active approaches that encourage an early return to activity.

One of the reasons for this important change in the focus of treatment is that an active approach minimizes the potential for the problem to develop into a chronic pain syndrome, which is resistant to successful management. Chronic disability becomes increasingly dissociated from the original physical basis.[23,36,56,57] An early return to activity as a result of restoration and improvement of function should be combined with biomechanical counseling that educates the patient in ways to remain active while still minimizing the potential for reinjury. This treatment direction helps to lessen

the possibility for the conversion of low back pain into low back disability and appears to be the future direction of successful management. Optimal treatment is now recognized as early and safe return to work and to activities of daily living.[43]

As a result of this further understanding, the low back dilemma has been reexamined. We must acknowledge that currently there are few methods of localizing the exact source of low back pain. There is also a paucity of controlled trials that allow for a determination of the most effective forms of management. Despite these shortcomings, the advances made in the natural and social sciences can and should be applied to managing the patient with low back pain.

MECHANICAL DISORDERS OF THE MUSCULOSKELETAL SYSTEM: MANAGEMENT PHILOSOPHIES

The previously stated new directions have resulted in a changing philosophy regarding the approaches to assessment and treatment of mechanical low back disorders. These changes parallel the approach to management of many mechanical disorders in other areas of the musculoskeletal system. Clinical practice for mechanical disorders can be briefly defined as an exercise in: (1) identifying the mechanics of injury, (2) recognizing the status of the injury, (3) maximizing the potential for repair processes of the musculoskeletal tissues, and (4) restoring function as rapidly as possible without reinjury in order to allow for functional healing.

This basic tenet of assessment and treatment has been the standard of care for extremity joints, but it has not been as well accepted for the low back. In no other area of the body is there such a plethora of traditional and nontraditional evaluation and treatment techniques. As a result, many patients develop a dependency on therapeutic interventions for symptomatic relief of low back pain at a much greater frequency than for any of the peripheral joints.

For example, the patient with an extremity

joint injury is usually expected to alter his activities in order to avoid exacerbation of the problem. Many times he must accept the fact that this alteration of activities must be maintained for the rest of his life. He is aware of his limitations and attempts to manage his own problem.

Many patients with mechanical low back pain behave differently, however, partly because of how the "system" treats them. They expect the therapeutic interventions to "cure" their back pain. These patients develop the thought process that the injured state of their low back is not really their problem, but rather the clinician's or system's problem.

As a result of this type of thinking, "quick cures" are continually sought after by the clinician and patient alike: modalities to "heal" tissue, manipulation to free "locked" joints or "trapped" structures, mobilization to "release" soft tissues, surgery to "reconstruct" the low back anatomy along a perceived normal, and specialty exercise devices designed to "eliminate" pain.

These examples of treatment, and others with similar intent, are successful in only a small number of select patients, and have little impact on the long-range outcome. These techniques alter the patient's perception of pain, rather than restore his function. It is thought that if the pain is "taken away," function will automatically return. In most cases these approaches are temporary solutions at best because the patient is not taught how to manage his own problem. What was once pain now becomes disability.

Contrast this with current methods of management for knee injury. Evaluation of the knee problem and therapeutic interventions to treat it are designed to restore function and teach the person the limits of activity. No matter what the therapeutic intervention, the desired outcome is increased function. A patient with a ligament injury, for example, accepts that he may have to modify his activity because his function will probably not be at the same level that it was before the injury.

Why is the approach to managing a knee injury different than the approach to managing low back pain? Certainly there are many answers and opinions. A case can be made, however, for the inability of the clinician to determine the exact source of pain in most low back pain syndromes. Additionally, many patients are unable to maximize their healing potential by using the same methods that have traditionally been successful in the management of extremity injuries. These include such strategies as remaining non-weight-bearing or using splints to render an area much less vulnerable to reinjury. In other words, the principles and techniques used to optimize tissue repair capabilities and gradually restore function to allow injured tissue to heal along appropriate stress lines are used differently and are more difficult to apply with low back disorders.

Treatment of the low back problem is changing, however, in a manner that more closely parallels the advances made in anatomy, biomechanics, and exercise physiology, coupled with an understanding of soft tissue healing. New knowledge currently available allows us to understand the spine in ways not formerly appreciated. As we understand the structure and function in greater detail, new methods to maximize the healing process and restore function surface. Treatment of the low back region can begin to approach the same practicality as treatment of the extremity.

The intent of this text is to integrate these sciences, relative to the lumbopelvic region, in a manner that invites a logical progression of assessment and treatment. It is readily apparent that passive therapeutic modalities and multiple surgical interventions are not effective in the long-term management of the problem. Prolonged rest and passive physical therapy modalities no longer have a place in the treatment of the chronic problem.[41] The successful clinician of the future will be one who can guide the patient through a rehabilitation process that most quickly and safely restores function.

INJURY AND REPAIR

In order to have a basis that provides direction for assessment and treatment, it is important to understand the consequences of tissue injury, the repair processes, and the biomechanics of the musculoskeletal tissues relative to these processes. A basic premise of this text is that, like the peripheral joints, the soft tissues as well as the cartilaginous and bony tissues of the spine have the potential to be injured. Although certainly not a novel thought, the concept of the soft tissues of the spine as a source of pain caused by injury is not as readily accepted as in the case of soft tissue injuries in the peripheral joints. Lesions of the intervertebral disc and the degenerative bony changes seen with the aging process are more typically considered the primary sources of mechanical low back pain than are the musculoskeletal tissues. Indeed, herniated nucleus pulposus and degenerative joint disease are two of the most common ones given for injuries to the low back.

Injury can be defined as the acute damage to or loss of cells and intracellular matrix; repair is defined as the replacement of damaged or lost cells and extracellular matrix with new cells and matrices.[59] Regeneration is a repair process in which new tissue that is structurally and functionally identical to the normal tissue is produced.[59] There are other repair processes that result in the formation of tissue that is not identical to the injured tissue.[54] Also, many different tissues are related to the spine and, based on these operational definitions, any can sustain injury. Each tissue in turn has the potential to be repaired by mechanisms unique to its cellular composition and individual biochemistry.

Many factors come into play in order to determine whether the repair process will be of the regeneration type, or whether the injured tissue will need to be replaced with a dissimilar tissue. Two of the major factors that influence the result of this repair process are the availability of vascular supply and the extent of the injury. Tissues that are not typically thought of as having repair potential can undergo successful regeneration if the injury is sufficiently small. For example, muscle defects less than 3 g or articular cartilage defects less than 1 mm can successfully regenerate.[59]

However, injuries may occur in which the capacity for tissue regeneration is exceeded. In these instances the repair process for injured tissue results in the formation of a connective tissue scar. Replacement at the injury site with this type of tissue might be adequate in *approximating* the function of the tendon or ligament, but it will not be adequate for restoring the function of injured muscle, cartilage, or nerve tissue.

The healing process for tissues of the body typically begins with an inflammatory stage, followed by a second stage that entails cell and matrix proliferation, which forms a type of vascularized granulation tissue. During the second stage collagen is synthesized and is initially distributed in a random pattern. Subsequent stages result in remodeling and maturation of the collagen to form a connective tissue scar, which completes the repair process.[54] Connective tissue is thus vitally important in the repair processes of the musculoskeletal soft tissues.

Connective tissue is also an integral part of the noninjured musculoskeletal tissues. The mechanical properties are such that it is extensively used in both the movement and the stabilization demands of the musculoskeletal system. For these reasons a closer analysis of connective tissue is warranted.

CONNECTIVE TISSUE

There are many types of basic tissues in the human body. Tissues are formed by cooperating cells that are assembled in coherent associations, and are bound together by fibrous and amorphous intercellular substances.[9] The basic tissues of the body include epithelium, connective tissue, blood, muscle tissue, adipose tissue, and nervous tissue. Of particular interest for understanding mechanical disorders are the structure and function of connective tissue and muscle tissue, and the interrelations between the two.

Structure

Connective tissue can be divided into connective tissue proper and the highly specialized connective tissue subclasses. Connective tissue proper can be further subdivided into

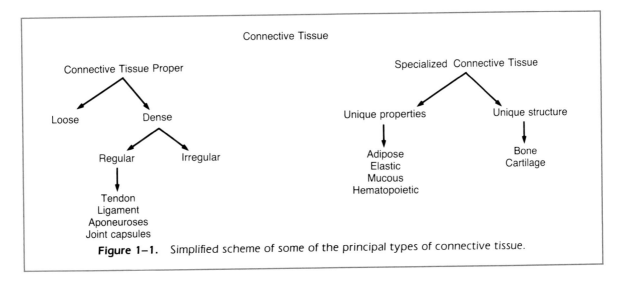

Figure 1–1. *Simplified scheme of some of the principal types of connective tissue.*

loose or dense connective tissue. Examples of dense connective tissue include tendon and ligament, and the specialized subclasses include cartilage and bone (Fig. 1–1). Despite the uniqueness of each type of connective tissue, they can be grouped under one family because of the similarity of the building blocks.

Connective tissues contain various concentrations of cells imbedded in an extracellular matrix. The matrix is composed of fibers and a ground substance. It is the distinct type of cell and the biochemical properties of the matrix that distinguish the type of connective tissue. Different types of proteins are synthesized by the cells and exist in various forms within the matrix. This determines the properties of the connective tissue. For example, the rigid structure of bone, the resiliency of cartilage, and the ability of connective tissue proper to yield are dependent on the aggregation of glycosaminoglycans and proteins to form the ground substance within the extracellular matrix.

Three types of fibers are seen in the various connective tissues: collagen, elastin, and reticulin. Collagen is the most abundant fiber type and has been further classified into subclasses.[20,39] The type of collagen synthesized is related to the specialized function of the connective tissue.

The orientation of the collagen also plays an important role in determining the function of the connective tissue. For example, the parallel arrangement of the collagen fibers, densely packed together, allows for the force of muscle contraction to be transmitted into and through the skeletal system with minimal elongation of the tendon. Because the tendon resists this deformation, it can be said that it has a certain stiffness. If the tendon lacked this stiffness, the force of muscle contraction would be diminished as it reached the bone. By comparison, the collagen of ligament is less highly ordered than tendon, yet its structural framework provides stiffness—resistance to deformation—to minimize movements in some directions while still allowing for movements in others.

The building block of collagen is tropocollagen, which consists of three polypeptide chains arranged in a triple helix (Fig. 1–2). The cross-linking of tropocollagen units enables collagen to have its great mechanical strength. Of particular importance in understanding the mechanics of the connective tissues is the wave-like undulations of the collagen fiber. This undulating phenomenon is known as "crimp."

Biomechanics

The crimp of the collagen is one of the major factors behind the viscoelastic response of connective tissue and the characteristics of the

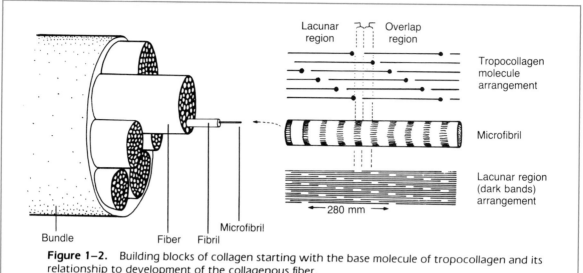

Figure 1–2. Building blocks of collagen starting with the base molecule of tropocollagen and its relationship to development of the collagenous fiber.

stress–strain curve (Fig. 1–3). It is thought to give the connective tissue a type of elasticity so that a structure such as a ligament behaves as a stiff spring as the crimp is straightened out by

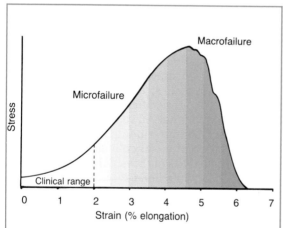

Figure 1–3. Stress/strain curve showing the amount of change and force imparted to collagenous structures. As a tensile force is imparted to the collagenous structure, the fibers straighten out or decrease the "crimp" (toe phase). As the force continues, the fibers arrange themselves in the lines of the force. Microtrauma results as the force continues until failure at approximately 6 to 8 per cent of elongation.

application of load.[25] The crimp is different for each kind of connective tissue, and consequently each tissue has a unique viscoelastic property.

The stress–strain curve graphically depicts the behavior of connective tissue as a stress is applied to the tissue. The curve starts with the toe region. In this range the connective tissue deforms easily, without the need for excessive force. The next region is the linear region, which represents the elastic stiffness of the connective tissue. If the applied forces are kept within this range, the tissue returns to its original shape. In this region crimp plays an important role. However, if the application of force increases beyond a certain point in the linear region, microtears of the tissue result. Finally, the stress–strain curve shows a rapid drop to zero if the force is further increased, and this represents failure of the connective tissue.

The biomechanics of connective tissue are important to consider because of the implications for injury. If the stress applied to the tissue is such that it exceeds the viscoelastic properties of the tissue, tissue failure results. This failure can be in the form of microscopic tears to the tissue or complete rupture of the tissue.

However, it is not only the strength of the

collagen fiber that is important, but also the condition of the intercellular matrix. The collagen interacts with the ground substance to form a concentration proportional to the viscoelastic needs required by the specific tissue. The ground substance contains mucopolysaccharides in the form of glycosaminoglycan that aggregate with proteins to determine the viscosity of the ground substance. The protein–glycosaminoglycan structure, known as a proteoglycan, is one of the most important factors in maintaining the normal function of the tissues. Therefore, it is not only a change in the nature of the collagen, but also any change in the matrix that ultimately determines the viscoelastic properties of the tissue.

Because each type of connective tissue and specialized connective tissue has a unique allocation and arrangement of collagen, proteoglycans, and water, the stress–strain curve is different for each tissue. Likewise, the same type of connective tissue (i.e., two ligaments from different areas) will show a difference in the stress–strain curve. The difference is due to the uniquely ordered structural matrix of each ligament, which depends on the area in which it is located and the stresses it must withstand.

All connective tissues, therefore, have unique structural properties that help to determine the functional capabilities and limitations of the tissue. Scar tissue, which is a form of specialized connective tissue, also displays properties that are different from the original tissue being replaced. These properties in turn result in altered function of the injured tissue.

In order to have a reference point from which to speculate as to the potential impact of tissue injury, it is appropriate to select some of the specialized tissues and briefly discuss their function. With an understanding of normal structure and function, the result of injury to the tissues can be better appreciated. Although a detailed account of the structure and function of individualized tissues is beyond the scope of this book, some salient points are addressed in order to allow for the formulation of hypotheses concerning the assessment and management of mechanical disorders of the musculoskeletal system. These concepts can then be applied toward an understanding of lumbopelvic disorders.

LIGAMENTS AND JOINT CAPSULE

Ligaments and joint capsules typically consist of an array of closely packed collagen fibers that allow for their classification as dense connective tissue. Their fibrous composition allows for stabilization of the joints. They are also flexible and allow for joint movement. Because of the location of the ligaments and capsules and the directions of their fibers, motion can be restricted in one direction while ample movement is possible in another. Thus the varied directions of joint motion are due in part to the orientation of the capsules and ligaments.

Ligaments and joint capsules function not only as support tissue, but also as a source of afferent input to the central nervous system. The importance of afferent feedback from these structures has been recognized, especially in regard to initiating reflex activity of the musculature.[16,27,35,46,62] In recent years Skinner and Barrack,[5,6,48,49] in a series of eloquent studies, have advanced our knowledge of the neurosensory role of the ligaments. Although caution must be taken to extrapolate their work to the low back, their results show conclusively that some ligaments can play a major role in providing afferent stimulus to the central nervous system, and loss of this neural input owing to ligament injury significantly diminishes a person's proprioceptive capabilities.[6]

Therefore, ligaments can no longer be viewed as passive structures, but as important components of the reflex systems. Further research is necessary to quantify the influence that the receptors of the lumbar and sacroiliac joint capsules, as well as the receptors within the numerous support ligaments, have on motor control of the lumbopelvic region. It can only be speculated that significant damage to these connective tissue structures caused by low back injury results in altered proprioceptive input, which in turn leads to a modification of movement patterns.

Although repair processes are discussed below, it is important to note that because the ligament and capsule are a fairly thick connective tissue structure of specific length, the outcome from repair processes depends not only on the strength of tissue, but on the length of the newly repaired tissue as well. If the repaired ligament or capsule does not return to its appropriate length, then this laxity impedes the ability to stabilize joint motion. Additionally, the repairing ligament or capsule that is immobilized too long results in the opposite ligament length problem—one of excessive stiffness. In both cases the outcome is either a lack of shortening of the ligament or excessive shortening of the ligament. Both processes alter joint mechanics and neural input. Combined, these have a potential effect on motor output.

ARTICULAR CARTILAGE

Articular cartilage is a highly specialized class of connective tissue with distinctive properties. It has a very high tensile strength and is resistant to compressive and shearing forces. At the same time it possesses some resilience and elasticity. The surface of articular cartilage is extremely smooth and relatively wear-resistant, and when combined with synovial fluid, it provides an exceptionally low coefficient of friction between articulating surfaces. As with the other classes of connective tissue, it is the arrangement and types of specific proteoglycans, collagens, and cells, in association with water, that determine the properties of cartilage. A change in one of the structural components will alter articular cartilage function, and thus its capacity to accept the various stresses placed on it.

Proteoglycans contribute between 30 per cent and 35 per cent of the dry weight of cartilage.[42] They form the major macromolecule of the cartilage ground substance. The type of proteoglycans and the manner in which they are aggregated are important to the structural rigidity of the extracellular matrix. In addition, the viscoelastic properties of cartilage depend on the concentration of proteoglycans in solution.[59]

There is now good evidence that the structure and composition of the proteoglycans in articular cartilage change with age.[12] Because proteoglycans are important for maintaining cartilage stiffness, especially in regard to compression, and also contribute to the resilience of cartilage, an alteration in proteoglycan composition reduces these qualities.[31] This in turn alters the biomechanics of articular cartilage.

Articular cartilage contains different types of collagen (Fig. 1–4). The properties of collagen provide the tissue with its tensile stiffness and strength. Type II collagen predominates, just as it does in normal nucleus pulposus. It is the combination of type II collagen in relation to proteoglycans that allows for and maintains an extremely high hydrated state, and thus makes this type of tissue well suited for compression stresses. The loading and unloading of the synovial joints squeeze water out of and back into the cartilage, and the removal of pressure rehydrates it.[30]

This rehydration phenomenon contributes to the nutrition of the cartilage as well by the changeover of fluid content. Although cartilage is described as an avascular structure, this is not entirely correct. What is actually meant is that the chondrocytes are located at a greater distance from the circulation as compared with other tissues.[58] Because of this vascular limitation, the contribution by rehydration is important in maintaining the health of the chondrocyte.

Chondrocyte health is important to consider because this cell is responsible for the existence and maintenance of the cartilage matrix. It is not known what signals the chondrocyte uses to alter the matrix. Understanding how the chondrocyte is signaled holds great promise in providing some of the answers related to cartilage repair.

MUSCLE TISSUE

The structure and function of muscle is reviewed in Chapter 3. However, it is also important to briefly discuss muscle at this time with regard to injury. Muscle is a highly specialized tissue that has an elaborately organized vascular and nerve supply. Because of this high degree of specialization, extensive injuries of muscle cannot be adequately regenerated to original muscle tissue. If regeneration cannot occur, muscle atrophy, rather than fibrous tissue replacement or scarring, results.[59]

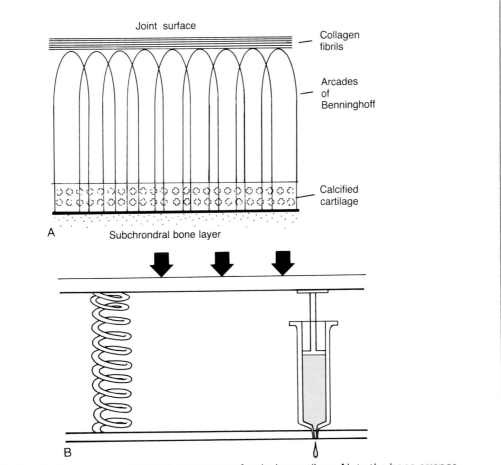

Joint surface

Collagen fibrils

Arcades of Benninghoff

Calcified cartilage

A   Subchrondral bone layer

B

Figure 1–4. *A,* A drawing depicting the structure of articular cartilage. Note the hoop arrangement of the middle layers of collagen. This structure permits function as shown in *B. B,* The mechanics of articular cartilage as shown in this sketch of a spring and syringe. As the cartilage is compressed, the descent is controlled by the hydraulics of the syringe and the rebound to normal height is dependent upon the spring. This permits shock absorption and also fluid movement needed to maintain health of the tissue.

If the muscle lesion is small enough, then the satellite cells, which are normally present between the basal lamina and the muscle fiber, differentiate into myoblasts to begin the process of muscle regeneration.[8,13] The myoblasts are myogenic cells that fuse to form myotubules. Through a gradual process, differentiation into muscle fibers ultimately occurs.[55]

A complete functional repair of muscle would necessarily include restoration of the previous innervation pattern, including motor nerve supply and sensory innervation from the muscle proprioceptors. Because normal muscle function also includes the development of appropriate vascular supply, this also becomes an important factor in determining whether the repair is complete. The restoration of muscle function after injury is critical because muscles are the motors that work with the fascial layers to direct the forces of weight-bearing and movement to bone and articular cartilage.

THE ATTENUATION OF TRUNK AND GROUND FORCES

With this brief overview of the structure and function of selected musculoskeletal tissues, we can speculate how they work collectively to counteract the forces of weight-bearing and movement. The center of gravity in the human body lies just anterior to the second sacral vertebrae in the erect, standing posture. By analyzing the anatomical adaptations that have occurred in response to the development of the upright posture, the lumbopelvic region can rightfully be viewed as a hub of weight-bearing. Hub refers to a region into which trunk and ground forces converge and are attenuated by the musculoskeletal tissues. In later chap-

ters the anatomy is described in detail and functional implications are discussed, but suffice it to say at this point that the lumbopelvic tissues appear to be extremely well designed for the maintenance of the upright posture.

What is meant by trunk and ground forces (Fig. 1–5)? The weight line of the head and trunk represent the trunk force component as it travels inferiorly into the lumbopelvic region. The ground reaction forces are those forces generated as a result of the establishment of a closed kinetic chain when the lower extremity comes in contact with the ground. These forces are directed superiorly into the lumbopelvic region. The musculoskeletal tissues, including those of the lumbopelvic region, function by either transferring the forces to the surrounding tissues or directly absorbing the forces. Each musculoskeletal tissue functions differently, but it is the combined interactions of these tissues that permit the desired outcome.

Each person is a combination of three basic

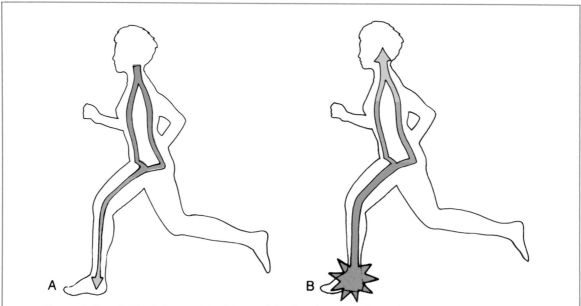

Figure 1–5.   A, Trunk forces. The forces of the head and trunk as they are transferred inferior into and through the actual skeleton. B, Ground forces as they are generated from the ground up through the actual skeleton into the trunk. The body has shock-absorbing and shock-transferring mechanisms that permit the proper transference of these forces.

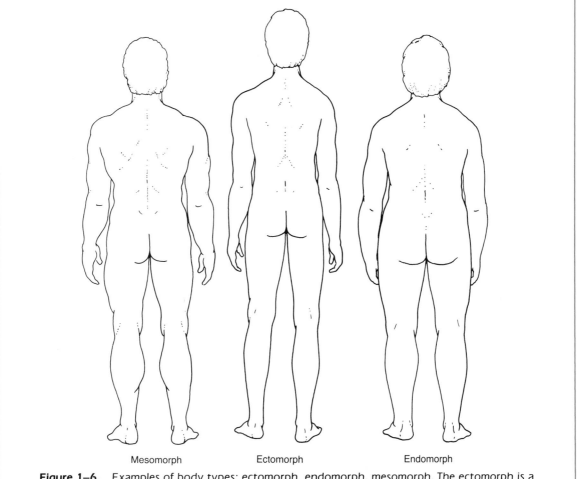

Figure 1–6. *Examples of body types: ectomorph, endomorph, mesomorph. The ectomorph is a long, lean individual. The endomorph has difficulty in managing body fat and has an abundance of fatty tissue. The mesomorph is generally muscular. We are all combinations of these three body types.*

Mesomorph   Ectomorph   Endomorph

body types: ectomorph, endomorph, and mesomorph (Fig. 1–6).[11] The predominant ectomorph is the person who is long and lean, and seldom varies from his body weight. His anthropometric features show a predominance of linearity and a relative fragility of body fluid, for example, the body type of the typical long-distance runner.

The predominant endomorph has a larger percentage of body fat, and has a difficult time maintaining a consistent body weight. His an-

thropometric features are more of corpulence and roundness. These people normally possess a great deal of joint mobility and are not as effective at sustaining the trunk and ground forces. We speculate that this lack of proper force transmission renders the supporting structures, especially the ligamentous tissue, vulnerable to injury. As a result, this population is usually not as active in those activities that require the dispersement of large super-incumbent and ground forces. When injured, this population can potentially have increased mobility and present with instability problems in the weight-bearing structures.

The person whose body type is predominantly mesomorphic has a relative predominance of muscularity, and less flexibility than the ectomorph. He does not readily attenuate the forces of gravity and movement, but quickly transfers these forces through tissues. We speculate that people with this body type have the potential to overload the bony matrix and strain the stiffer connective tissues with excessive activity. The ground force is poorly dampened as it moves through the foot, ankle, knee, hip, and spinal regions. The mesomorph presents a different clinical picture, for example, than the predominant endomorph, in that bony injury and frequent strains are more prominent. The mesomorph is more active, but generates forces that reach the physiologic limits of the optimal loading curve more quickly, with potential tissue breakdown as a result.

The analysis of body type is subjective. Most people have a body type that is represented along the continuum of all three body types. However, anthropometric features are an important clinical consideration in analyzing mechanical disorders of the musculoskeletal system. The relative body type of the patient must be identified because this information permits the clinician to make a judgment as to the manner in which the forces are passed through the region during the stresses of injury. As a "crossroads" of trunk and ground forces, the musculoskeletal tissues of the lumbopelvic region are vulnerable to sprain and strain injuries because they control the hub of weight-bearing. The tissues must respond appropriately to the demands of the activity without being damaged.

TISSUE RESPONSES TO STRESS

Tissues of the musculoskeletal system have a common denominator: they all require the stimulus of nondestructive stresses to maintain their health. Nondestructive stresses refer to activities that result in the stresses of movement and weight-bearing within the physio-

logic limits of the musculoskeletal tissues. For example, cartilage nutrition,[43] muscle strength,[21] the strength of ligaments and their bony attachments,[1,52,53] and tensile strength of tendon[53,61] are all promoted with increased activity. Changes that improve the resilience of connective tissue structures include an increase in the diameter of collagen fiber bundles, higher collagen content,[51,52] and an increase in the ultimate load capabilities of tendons secondary to changes at the bone insertion sites.[61] This underscores the importance of the interaction between muscle tissue and its connective tissue counterparts.

It is safe to assume that one of the contributing factors to maintaining musculoskeletal health is activity that places controlled stresses on these tissues. Exactly *how* these stresses provide the signal for cellular activity that results in such effects as increased fibril size, connective tissue stiffness, and tissue strength is not known.

By comparison, immobilization has deleterious effects on the musculoskeletal tissues. Changes include loss of water content, altered proteoglycan concentrations, and a decreased overall strength of the tissue. As a result, deterioration of cartilage, tendons, ligaments, and muscle occurs.[2,10,14,19,38]

Figure 1–7 shows the concept of optimal versus destructive loading patterns of musculoskeletal tissues. As implied with the graph, there is an optimal loading range of tissues that helps to maintain the health of the tissue. This is represented by the middle portion of the graph. When the various forces of weight-bearing and movement, coupled with the forces exerted by way of muscle contraction, remain within the optimal loading range, the health of the tissue is assured.

Conversely, as mentioned above, musculoskeletal tissues weaken from overuse or disuse. If the forces to the tissues exceed the upper limit of the optimal loading zone, tissue breakdown destruction results. This destructive stimulus can come in the form of a single high-impact load, like that experienced with a fall or a motor vehicle accident. For example, Donahue and associates[17] noted that impact loading to articular cartilage can not only result in fracture of the cartilage, but also cause cartilage

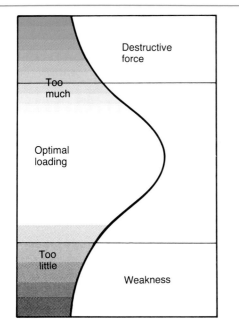

Figure 1–7. A bell-shaped curve placed on its side depicting the concept of optimal loading patterns and destructive loading patterns, both representing too much force and too little force. This is an example of specific adaptation to imposed demand (SAID).

swelling and a change in the proteoglycan and collagen association in the cartilage matrix. Potential tissue destruction occurs because the upper limit of the optimal loading zone has been reached.

Tissue breakdown may also occur with prolonged, excessive overloading, such as seen with overtraining. Muscle fiber necrosis has been demonstrated after conditions of intense training and prolonged activity.[29,32] The accumulation of microstresses over a period of time breaks down muscle tissue.

Another example of overloading might occur with prolonged, asymmetrical stresses. In these instances the magnitude of the force is not as important as the length of time that the force is being applied. The repetitive stresses result in an accumulation of microscopic insults to the tissue. The long-term articular cartilage changes in one compartment of the knee after unilateral meniscectomy of that same com-

partment are a well-known example. After the meniscectomy the loading patterns of the knee joint articular cartilage are altered, and degeneration patterns such as articular cartilage damage and subchondral bone changes result.[15,18,47] Frontal plane asymmetry leading to asymmetrical loading patterns of the hips results in degenerative changes of the articular cartilage of the hip joint.[28] The various stresses to the soft tissue of the spine with asymmetrical loading patterns are described later in this text.

OPTIMAL LOADING ZONE ALTERATION

The optimal loading zone shown in Figure 1–7 can be altered over a period of time by three main factors (Fig. 1–8). The first is *age*. With the aging process there is change in both the type and the aggregation patterns of proteoglycans. The tissues change both structurally and functionally as we age. For example, in articular cartilage, chondroitin sulfate content decreases and the aggregations of proteoglycans become smaller.[12] These changes alter the water-binding capacity of the molecule, and thus its shock-attenuating capacity.

Changes in the proteoglycan and collagen makeup also affect the properties of the soft tissues. Factors known to influence structural and mechanical properties of ligaments and their insertions are age and mechanical stress.[59] Because of age-related changes, the matrix becomes more fibrous and the viscosity is increased. This in turn alters the mobility and failure rate of the tissues. These do not represent the only changes of the aging process, however; aging ultimately decreases the ability of the tissue to withstand the magnitude and duration of forces that were formerly tolerated.

The second factor that alters the upper limit of the optimal loading zone is *adaptive change*. A clinical example might best demonstrate this phenomenon. The person who leads a sedentary life-style exhibits structural adaptive changes over the course of many years. He may

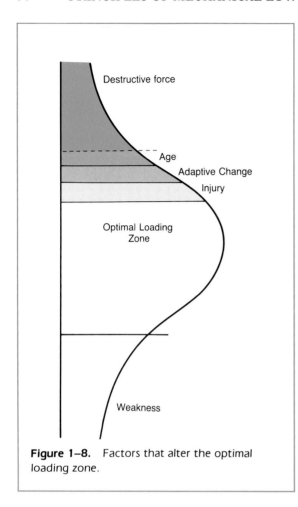

Figure 1–8. Factors that alter the optimal loading zone.

develop shortened hamstring and anterior hip muscles and tight hip joint capsules from prolonged sitting, and a weakened or stretched abdominal wall. These structural changes can be added to body composition changes that also occur. The average person gains 1 lb of total body weight per year and loses 1 per cent of muscle strength per year after age 25.[63] This further accentuates the adaptation of the musculoskeletal tissues.

When this person presents to the clinician with the first episode of low back pain, he does not often relate the physical changes over the past years as the precursor to the mechanical disorder giving rise to pain. Rather, the focus is on the single episode that initiated the painful syndrome. Adaptive changes in the form of connective tissue shortening and muscle weakness reduce the musculoskeletal system's tolerance to stresses. Recognition of these changes is important because they influence the treatment approach. This point is discussed more fully in Chapters 5 and 6.

The third factor that alters the loading capacity of the tissues is *injury*. After the musculoskeletal tissue is damaged, healing begins. As this process continues, the end result is repair with a tissue related in structure but different from the original tissue that was damaged.

The repair process, however, does not typically restore the tissue to its former capacity. As an example, after injury to the medial collateral ligament of the knee, the tensile strength returns to only 50 per cent to 70 per cent of the original, preinjured tensile strength.[26,60] There is no reason to suspect that ligamentous healing in the lumbopelvic region is markedly different. Indeed, it may be even harder to develop a strong, functional repair, since it is difficult to immobilize this region with the same efficacy as the shoulder or knee joint. Because of the convergence of trunk and ground forces in the lumbopelvic region, this area is vulnerable to multiple stresses. It can be speculated that the stages of repair will proceed, provided that destructive stimuli are kept from the area. One of the keys to management is to minimize the chances for these destructive stimuli to reach the region. Significant injuries can ultimately result in permanent impairment, which can lead to adaptive changes, recurring pain, and loss of function.

Age and injury also influence the proprioceptive activity in the musculoskeletal tissues. Because some of the receptors are highly specialized connective tissue structures themselves, injury to the ligament, tendon, or joint capsule might also damage the receptor. Additionally, as a person ages, the number of proprioceptors related to the tissues decreases. The combination of these changes probably alters the afferent input to the central nervous system.

These three factors (age, adaptive changes, and injury) alter musculoskeletal tissue tolerance to stresses. As a result, a stimulus that was formerly nondestructive to the area may now be destructive or injurious. There is, in effect, a new and now lowered maximal limit of tissue tolerance.

The lower end of the graph depicted in Figure 1–7 remains relatively consistent in its position. As mentioned above, it is recognized that if the tissues of the musculoskeletal system do not have physiologic stresses applied to them, they undergo degenerative changes. This results in weaker tissue that is unable to properly attenuate forces, and predisposes the region to injury and the potential for the cyclic pattern of injury-pain-reinjury.

So the critical issue is determining how much stress is too much, and how much exceeds the physiologic capacity for the musculoskeletal tissues. It is a well-accepted axiom that the tissues of the musculoskeletal system not only develop, but also heal in accordance with the stresses placed on them. Perhaps the most well-known example of this phenomenon is Wolff's law.[45] This law states that bone is laid down according to the stresses placed on it. Bone thickens at those points where the stresses are greatest and thins at the areas in which the load is diminished. The trabecular pattern forms as a result of the various compression and tensile forces imparted to the bone. Specialized cells—the osteoblast and the osteoclast—are available to carry out this task. Other tissues of the musculoskeletal system also respond to the same basic principle. For example, the connective tissues of the ligament, tendon, and matrix of muscle respond in the same manner to the stresses of activity by making the necessary adaptations to the increased demands.

Muscle tissue is also capable of making adaptations as a result of the stresses incurred. For example, muscle tissue changes both anatomically and biochemically in response to demands placed on it. Endurance training increases the capacity of the mitochondria to generate adenosine triphosphate aerobically by oxidative phosphorylation, and also increases the number and size of the mitochondria.[40] This is a response to the type of training demands placed on the muscle. Even the skin follows this basic principle of adaptation as it adapts to the frictional stresses of weight-bear-ing by forming a callus at that point where the overload occurred.

Essentially all of the musculoskeletal tissues respond to the various long-term stresses placed on them by adaptation. This response has been described as a specific adaptation to imposed demand (SAID).[4] The SAID principle is an acronym used to relate the effects of sports conditioning and training. It indicates that conditioning and training are directed toward the specific demands of a given sport. It is an important concept because it provides a basis for the rehabilitation of most musculoskeletal disorders, and does not necessarily have to be limited to sports. The goal with rehabilitation programs for mechanical disorders is to prepare the body for the various stresses it may face. It is not exercise per se that results in a "cure." Instead, rehabilitation programs that emphasize activity (a form of musculoskeletal training) after the adaptations necessary to meet imposed demands. Later in the text the concept of training is discussed in its rehabilitation context. Suffice it to say at this point that when the adaptations in response to training occur, a more active life-style becomes a reachable goal.

Therefore, the clinician's goal in the management of mechanical disorders is to identify the injury status of the tissues and provide a treatment plan designed to do the following:

1. Optimize the environment to heal the wound
2. Maintain the relations of the injured tissues to the noninjured tissues
3. Maintain the health of the noninjured tissues
4. Place nondestructive forces that will assure functional healing to the injured tissues
5. Prevent the application of excessive forces to the injured tissues

Although these objectives are more fully explored in Chapter 6, they should be mentioned in the context of the SAID principle. Understanding the SAID principle is especially important in regard to number 4 above, and is one of the major reasons that a more active approach to managing mechanical low back disorders is preferred. The inability to effectively carry out this plan of care for a musculoskeletal tissue injury leads to various forms of tissue dysfunction, such as contracture, adhesion, laxity, and diminished function, and we speculate that it subsequently alters neurophysiologic feedback.

Mismanagement also results in frequent reinjury, mainly because of the dysfunction of the region, and chronic symptoms. Prevention of the syndrome, and, more important, prevention of disability from a mechanical low back disorder, is facilitated by prompt, accurate identification of the injury and the beginning of a goal-oriented, supervised rehabilitation program. These types of programs are best designed by a professional who is skilled in the analysis of human movement, recognizes the three-dimensional relations of anatomical structures, and understands the processes of tissue healing.

✳CAUSES OF MECHANICAL LOW BACK PAIN

When causes of low back pain are discussed, it is usually the structure that is named rather than the etiology. For example, a partial list of the common causes of low back pain might include the intervertebral disc, zygapophyseal joints, bony elements, and the muscle.

Close inspection of this list reveals that these are not causative factors. We should think of the causes more in terms of sprains, strains, or structural failure. For example, a force applied to the outer annular ring of the intervertebral disc that exceeds the viscoelasticity of that tissue causes a permanent elongation of that structure. A sprain of an annular ring has occurred, and it no longer functions normally. This is much like the example of the knee joint injury in which the viscoelasticity of the anterior cruciate ligament is exceeded, and permanent elongation of the ligament results. The ligament has been sprained, and the manner in which forces are accepted by other tissues in the knee is now altered. The degenerative processes of the surrounding tissues are hastened. We can safely assume that the sprained annulus fibrosus will also alter the normal force acceptance in the lumbopelvic region.

This alteration of mechanics owing to injury is the case with any tissue in the lumbopelvic region. The biomechanics of this region require an interplay of multiple joints, especially the lumbar zygapophyseal, sacroiliac, and hip joints, their connective tissue restraining elements, and muscular effort at both a conscious and a reflex level. If the mechanical forces applied to the lumbopelvic region are not attenuated by these multiple tissues, then the mechanical threshold of the tissue may be exceeded. The rich nociceptive system in this region is then stimulated by mechanical deformation or chemical irritation of the nociceptors (see Chapter 2). It becomes vital to remove the offending force from this nociceptive system in order to control the painful syndrome and restore function.

Therefore, the concept that is to be presented in this text is that *it does not matter what tissue is involved in the cause of mechanical low back pain, but rather the abnormal or excessive force(s) that converge into the region that chemically and/or mechanically stimulate the nociceptive system and result in pain.*

We suggest that the alteration and attenuation of forces that remove nociceptive stimulation in the lumbopelvic unit might be a unifying element between the many and varied treatment techniques being used for low back pain. Reflex responses caused by modality or manual techniques may influence the central nervous system in such a way that the resultant response by the muscular system influences joint mechanics. Manual or surgical techniques attempt to remove an offending force or alter the way forces reach the area.

When viewed in this manner the "technique" becomes less important than the science. For this reason a major portion of this text is devoted to the three-dimensional aspects of the normal anatomy and the relations that tissues have with one another, both structurally and functionally. If the clinician has this understanding, then the assessment of the biomechanics of human movement can be more directly related to evaluation and treatment of mechanical low back pain.

Knowledge of mechanical low back disorders has matured beyond past notions that all back pain is from the intervertebral disc or the zygapophyseal joints, or is myofascial in nature, or that we often have only an isolated injury. If we can identify the offending forces, especially during a patient's activities of daily living, and minimize these forces while allowing the person to stay active, then the healing process will more readily occur. In effect, one of the goals of treatment for any mechanical injury is to provide an optimal healing environment.

The clinician and the patient are thus challenged to identify the forces that are stimulating the nociceptive system and reproducing symptoms, and to control and alter the way that they reach the lumbopelvic region. It is extremely important that the patient have an active role in this management. Less than 2 per cent of his waking time is spent in treatment. The clinician must convince the patient of the importance of the other 98 per cent of his waking time with respect to managing his own syndrome. Anything less invites failure and patient dependency on the health care professional. The clinician's responsibility is to understand the details of the functional anatomy of the region to allow for a purposeful evaluation and the development of a valid treatment protocol.

SUMMARY

In this chapter we briefly reviewed the important difference between low back pain and low back disability. As a hub of weight-bearing, the low back is susceptible to the various sprain, strain, and mechanical breakdowns as in the extremity joints. The response of the various tissues to injury and their subsequent repair processes are essentially the same whether they are in the low back or in the extremities. Therefore, the principles of evaluation and treatment should be similar.

The uniqueness of the lumbopelvic region is related to how the tissues respond to the convergence of trunk and ground forces. This in turn must be placed in the context of an optimal loading curve. When combined with a working knowledge of the functional anatomy of the region, a logical progression of evaluation and treatment can begin.

REFERENCES

1. Adams A: Effect of exercise upon ligament strength. Res Q 37:163, 1966.
2. Akeson WH, Woo SL-Y, Amiel D, et al: The connective tissue response to immobility: Biochemical changes in periarticular connective tissue of the immobilized rabbit knee. Clin Orthop 93:356, 1973.
3. Andersson GBJ: Epidemiologic aspects of lowback pain in industry. Spine 10:482, 1985.
4. Arnheim DD: Modern Principles of Athletic Training. St. Louis, C.V. Mosby, 1985.
5. Barrack RL, Skinner HB, Brunet ME, et al: Functional performance of the knee after intraarticular anesthesia. Am J Sports Med 11:258, 1983.
6. Barrack RL, Skinner HB, Buckley SL: Proprioception in the anterior cruciate deficient knee. Am J Sports Med 17:1, 1989.
7. Benn RT, Wood PHN: Pain in the back: An attempt to estimate the size of the problem. Rheumatol Rehabil 14:121, 1975.
8. Bischoff R: A satellite cell mitogen from crushed adult muscle. Dev Biol 115:140, 1986.
9. Bloom W, Fawcett DW: Textbook of Histology. Philadelphia, W.B. Saunders, 1975.
10. Bortz WM: The disuse syndrome. West J Med 141:691, 1984.
11. Brooks GA, Fahey TD: Exercise Physiology: Human Bioenergetics and Its Applications. New York, John Wiley & Sons, 1984.
12. Buckwalter JA, Kuettner KE, Thonar EJM: Age-related changes in articular cartilage proteoglycans: Electron microscopic studies. J Orthop Res 3:251, 1985.
13. Campion DR: The muscle satellite cell: A review. Int Rev Cytol 87:225, 1984.
14. Cooper RR: Alterations during immobilization and regeneration of skeletal muscle in cats. J Bone Joint Surg 54A:919, 1972.
15. Cox JS, Cordell LD: The degenerative effects of medial meniscus tears in dogs' knees. Clin Orthop 125:236, 1977.
16. Dee R: Structure and function of hip joint innervation. Ann R Coll Surg Engl 45:357, 1969.
17. Donahue JM, Buss D, Oegema TR, et al: The effects of indirect blunt trauma on adult canine articular cartilage. J Bone Joint Surg 65A:948, 1983.
18. Elmer RM, Moskowitz RW, Frankel VH: Meniscal regeneration and postmeniscectomy degenerative joint disease. Clin Orthop 125:304, 1977.
19. Enneking WF, Horowitz M: The intra-articular effects of immobilization on the human knee. J Bone Joint Surg 54A:973, 1972.
20. Eyre DR: Collagen: Molecular diversity in the body's protein scaffold. Science 207:1315, 1980.
21. Faulkner JA: New perspectives in training for maximum performance. JAMA 205:741, 1986.
22. Fordyce WE, Brockway JA, Bergman JA, Spengler D: Acute back pain: A control group comparison of behavioural vs. traditional management methods. J Behav Med 9:127, 1986.
23. Fordyce WE, Fowler RS, Lehmann JF, DeLateur BJ:

Some implications of learning in problems of chronic pain. J Chron Dis 21:179, 1968.

24. Fordyce WE, McMahan R, Rainwater G, et al: Pain complaint-exercise performance relationship in chronic pain. Pain 10:311, 1981.

25. Frank C, Amiel D, Woo SL-Y, et al: Normal ligament properties and ligament healing. Clin Orthop 196:15, 1985.

26. Frank C, Woo SL-Y, Amiel D, et al: Medial collateral ligament healing: A multidisciplinary assessment in rabbits. Am J Sports Med 11:379, 1983.

27. Freeman MAR, Wyke B: Articular reflexes at the ankle joint: An electromyographic study of normal and abnormal influences of ankle-joint mechano-receptors upon reflex activity in the leg muscles. Br J Surg 54:990, 1967.

28. Friberg O: Clinical symptoms and biomechanics of lumbar spine and hip joint in leg length inequality. Spine 8:643, 1983.

29. Friden J, Sjostrom M, Ekblom B: Myofibrillar damage following intense eccentric exercise in man. Int J Sports Med 4:170, 1983.

30. Gradisar IA, Porterfield JA: Articular cartilage. Top Geriatr Rehabil 4:1, 1989.

31. Harris ED Jr, Parker HG, Radin EL, et al: Effects of proteolytic enzymes on structural and mechanical properties of cartilage. Arthritis Rheum 15:497, 1972.

32. Hikida RS, Staron RS, Hagerman FC, et al: Muscle fiber necrosis associated with human marathon runners. J Neurol Sci 59:185, 1983.

33. Holbrook T, Grazier K, Kelsey J, Stauffer R: The Frequency of Occurrence Impact and Cost of Selected Musculoskeletal Conditions in the United States. American Academy of Orthopedic Surgeons, 1984.

34. Kelsey J, White AA: Epidemiology and impact of low-back pain. Spine 6:133, 1980.

35. Kennedy JC, Alexander IJ, Hayes KC: Nerve supply of the human knee and its functional importance. Am J Sports Med 10:329, 1982.

36. Loeser JD, Fordyce WE: Chronic pain. In Carr JE, Dengerink HA (eds): Behavioural Science in the Practice of Medicine. New York, Elsevier, 1983.

37. Mayer TG, Gatchel RJ: Functional Restoration of Spinal Disorders: The Sports Medicine Approach. Philadelphia, Lea & Febiger, 1988.

38. Mayer TG, Gatchel RJ, Kitchino N, et al: Objective assessment of lumbar function following industrial injury. Spine 10:482, 1985.

39. Mayne R, Irwin MH: Collagen types in cartilage. In Kuettner KE, Schleyerbach R, Hascall VC (eds): Articular Cartilage Biochemistry, p. 38. New York, Raven Press, 1986.

40. McArdle WD, Katch FI, Katch VL: Exercise Physiology: Energy, Nutrition, and Human Performance. Philadelphia, Lea & Febiger, 1986.

41. Mooney V: Where is the pain coming from? Presidential address for International Society for the Study of the Lumbar Spine. Spine 12:754, 1987.

42. Muir IHM: The chemistry of the ground substance of joint cartilage. In Sokoloff L (ed): The Joints and Synovial Fluid, vol. 2, p. 27. New York, Academic Press, 1980.

43. Nachemson A: Work for all, for those with low back pain as well. Clin Orthop 179:77, 1983.

44. Nordby E: Epidemiology and diagnosis in lowback injury. Occup Health Safety 50:38, 1981.

45. Salter R: Textbook of Disorders and Injuries of the Musculoskeletal System, 2nd ed. Baltimore, Williams & Wilkins, 1983.

46. Schultz RA, Miller DC, Kerr CS, et al: Mechanoreceptors in human cruciate ligaments: A histological study. J Bone Joint Surg 66A:1072, 1984.

47. Shapiro F, Glimcher MJ: Induction of osteoarthrosis in the rabbit knee joint: Histologic changes following meniscectomy and meniscal lesions. Clin Orthop 147:287, 1980.

48. Skinner HB, Barrack RL, Cook SD: Age-related decline in proprioception. Clin Orthop 184:208, 1984.

49. Skinner HB, Barrack RL, Cook SD, et al: Joint position sense in total arthroplasty. J Orthop Res 1:276, 1984.

50. Spengler D, Bigos S, Martin N, et al: Back injuries in industry: A retrospective study. Overview and cost analysis. Spine 11:241, 1986.

51. Stone MH: Implications for connective tissue and bone alterations resulting from resistance exercise training. Med Sci Sports Exerc 20 (Suppl):S162, 1988.

52. Tipton CM, James SL, Mergner W, et al: Influence of exercise on strength of medial collateral knee ligaments in dogs. Am J Physiol 218:894, 1970.

53. Tipton CM, Matthes RD, Maynard JA, et al: The influence of physical activity on ligaments and tendons. Med Sci Sports 7:165, 1975.

54. van der Muelen JCH: Present state of knowledge on processes of healing in collagen structures. Int J Sports Med 3:4, 1982.

55. Vracko R, Benditt EP: Basal lamina: The scaffold for orderly cell replacement: Observations on regeneration of injured skeletal muscle fibers and capillaries. J Cell Biol 55:406, 1972.

56. Waddell G: A new clinical model for the treatment of low-back pain. Spine 12:632, 1987.

57. Waddell G, Main CJ, Morris EW, et al: Chronic low-back pain, psychological distress and illness behaviour. Spine 9:209, 1984.

58. Williams PL, Warwick R: Gray's Anatomy, 36th Br. ed. Philadelphia, W.B. Saunders, 1986.

59. Woo SL-Y, Buckwalter JA: Injury and Repair of the Musculoskeletal Soft Tissues. American Academy of Orthopedic Surgeons, Park Ridge, Illinois, 1988.

60. Woo SL-Y, Inoue M, McGurk-Burleson E, et al: Treatment of the medial collateral ligament injury. II. Structure and function of canine knees in response to differing treatment regimens. Am J Sports Med 15:22, 1987.

61. Woo SL-Y, Ritter MA, Amiel D, et al: The effects of exercise on the biomechanical and biochemical properties of swine digital flexor tendons. J Biomech Eng 103:51, 1981.

62. Wyke B: Neurological aspects of low back pain. In Jayson M (ed): Lumbar Spine and Back Pain, p. 189. New York, Grune & Stratton, 1976.

63. Zarins B: Soft tissue injury and repair—biomechanical aspects. Int J Sports Med 3:9, 1982

2

NEUROMECHANICAL BASIS OF LUMBOPELVIC FUNCTION AND DYSFUNCTION

The complete field of neurosciences is certainly too large to be presented in a text of this nature. However, certain aspects of neurosciences, especially as they relate to mechanical disorders, can be applied to an understanding of lumbopelvic function and dysfunction. In everyday clinical practice, some aspect of neuroanatomy and neurophysiology is utilized in the evaluation and management of lumbopelvic problems. This chapter focuses on aspects of the neurosciences that are relevant to the phenomenon of mechanical low back disorders. In particular, the details of the nerve root complex, the innervation of lumbopelvic tissues, and the interaction between the sensory and motor aspects of motor behavior are discussed.

These three topics are chosen because of their relevance to the various etiology, evaluation, and treatment theories related to mechanical low back pain. For example, new knowledge of the anatomy and physiology of the lumbosacral nerve roots has allowed us to more completely understand the mechanisms that lead to nerve root (radicular) pain. In order to reinforce the importance of recognizing potential nerve root involvement, a neurologic screening examination for mechanical low back pain patients is also included in this chapter.

The innervation of the lumbopelvic tissues, and how the various elements of the nervous system are involved with motor control, has allowed us to recognize the synergistic behavior of the trunk and extremity musculature and the importance of the sensory system in movement patterns. Muscle is an effector organ because it converts neural commands into a desired force. This force contributes to movement or stability. In order to generate smooth, purposeful motor activity, information from the various sensory receptors must be channeled into the central nervous system in order to allow for an appropriate interaction between motor control centers and the activity of different muscles.

Mechanical low back pain alters this afferent-efferent balance, and in the broadest sense, many patients who suffer from low back pain can be viewed as having movement disorders. Various treatment regimens emphasize sensory stimulation, motor enhancement, or both. Their goal has been to improve neuromuscular efficiency to increase psychophysical outcomes. It is hoped that through the discourse on lumbopelvic innervation and the receptor system, common threads can be seen in the various treatment programs utilized for functional restoration of low back disability. This discussion of treatment is continued and detailed more thoroughly in Chapter 6.

In order to present the information in a manner that allows for clinical comments to be made at the same time that the structure and function are discussed, this chapter is organized according to the regional anatomy. Starting centrally, the nerve roots are discussed first. Moving laterally, the innervation of the lumbopelvic tissues with the associated rami and peripheral nerves is next addressed. Final consideration is given to the receptor system located peripherally in the tissues themselves.

THE NERVE ROOTS

After Mixter and Barr's[41] report in 1934, the nerve root and its relation to the intervertebral disc received great attention. The results of that study were interpreted as demonstrating that the major mechanism behind the clinical syndromes of low back and leg pain was compression of the nerve roots by the protruded intervertebral disc.

In subsequent years research into the structure and function of the nerve root has led to a clearer understanding of its unique nature. In addition, the osseus and nonosseus tissues that surround it have also been more completely described. Recognition is now given to the fact that structures other than the disc can adversely influence the nerve roots in their path from the spinal canal to the intervertebral foramen. Detailed descriptions of the meningeal coverings, pedicle of the vertebrae, lateral recess, zygapophyseal joint, transforamenal ligaments, and the contents within the intervertebral foramen are now available, and have been investigated as to their potential influence on nerve root function. The purpose of this section is to detail the anatomy of the nerve root and the structures it interacts with along its course and then consider its role in low back pain.

The nerve roots are the motor and sensory pathways that link the central nervous system with the tissues and organs of the body. Because the spinal cord ends opposite the intervertebral disc between the second and third lumbar vertebrae, the nerve roots must be progressively longer in order to make their exit at the spinal level below their respective vertebrae.[2] In the lumbosacral region these elongated roots form the cauda equina, which traverse the lower lumbar vertebral spinal canal (Fig. 2–1). The obliquity of the course of the nerve roots gradually increases as we proceed inferiorly. The first and second lumbar nerve roots have an angle of inclination of 70 to 80 degrees; the third and fourth, 60 degrees; the fifth, 45 degrees; and the first sacral nerve root, 30 degrees.[6]

The nerve roots are formed by rootlets that are attached to the spinal cord, and converge to form the fibers of the root cylinder (Fig. 2–2). The fibers from these rootlets form the nerve roots in parallel bundles. The ventral nerve root and the typically larger dorsal nerve root then stream toward the intervertebral foramen. At the foramen the dorsal and ventral root merge to form the mixed spinal nerve (hereafter referred to as spinal nerve).[53] Just medial to this merging is the dorsal root ganglion, which is a distinct swelling located on the dorsal root. The dorsal root ganglion rep-

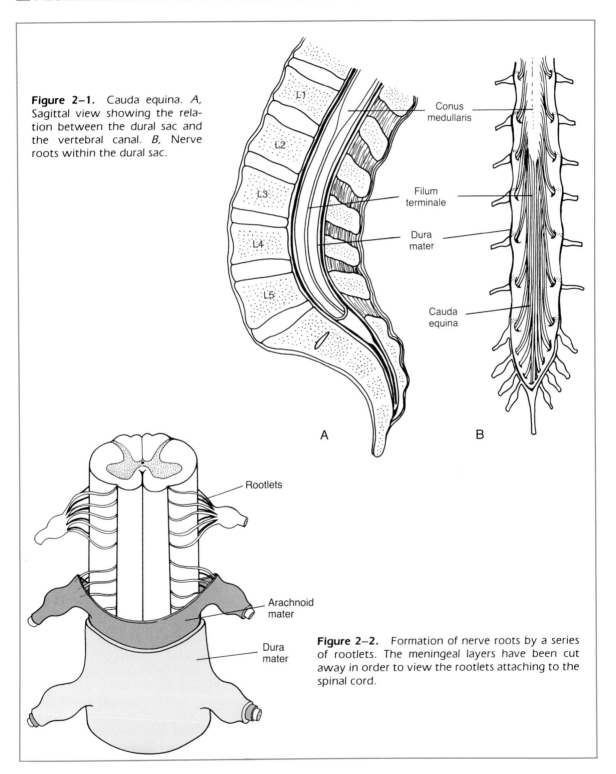

Figure 2–1. Cauda equina. *A*, Sagittal view showing the relation between the dural sac and the vertebral canal. *B*, Nerve roots within the dural sac.

Conus medullaris

Filum terminale

Dura mater

Cauda equina

L1

L2

L3

L4

L5

A   B

Rootlets

Arachnoid mater

Dura mater

Figure 2–2. Formation of nerve roots by a series of rootlets. The meningeal layers have been cut away in order to view the rootlets attaching to the spinal cord.

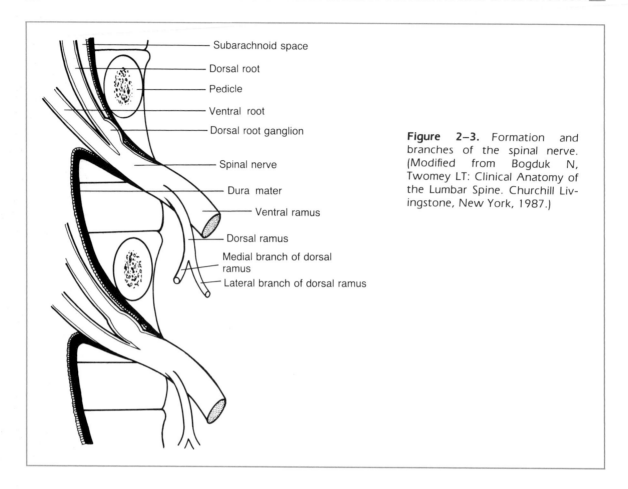

Subarachnoid space
Dorsal root
Pedicle
Ventral root
Dorsal root ganglion
Spinal nerve
Dura mater
Ventral ramus
Dorsal ramus
Medial branch of dorsal ramus
Lateral branch of dorsal ramus

Figure 2–3. Formation and branches of the spinal nerve. (Modified from Bogduk N, Twomey LT: Clinical Anatomy of the Lumbar Spine. Churchill Livingstone, New York, 1987.)

resents a cluster of cell bodies that give rise to the axons that actually form the dorsal nerve root. The spinal nerve continues through the intervertebral foramen and bifurcates, forming the dorsal and ventral rami, which continue into the tissues. The peripheral nerves then branch from the dorsal or ventral rami (Fig. 2–3).

AXOPLASMIC TRANSPORT AND NERVE ROOT FUNCTION: IMPLICATIONS FOR LOW BACK DYSFUNCTION

In their simplest description, all nerve roots, spinal nerves, rami, and peripheral nerves are organized bundles of cellular processes that extend from nerve cell bodies. These cellular processes are axon cylinders, also referred to as nerve fibers. The nerve cell bodies that give rise to these axon cylinders are located in the ventral horn of the spinal cord and in the dorsal root ganglion.[48] The name given to an axon cylinder (nerve root, spinal nerve, ramus, or peripheral nerve) is determined by the anatomical region in which that axon cylinder is located (Fig. 2–4).

The cell bodies of the dorsal root ganglion are anatomically unique structures in the nervous system, and deserve special mention. Although they appear to give rise to only one axon that bifurcates into two branches, they actually derive from bipolar cells whose two processes fused during embryologic development. One branch is the peripheral axon, which is attached to the receptors in the periphery, and the other is the central axon, which contributes to the formation of the dorsal root.[50]

The fact that the axon cylinder is a cellular extension of the nerve cell body is important to recognize in order to understand how the nerve cell provides the necessary neuronal proteins to the axon terminals. In addition, used materials can be returned to the cell body for either degradation or restoration and reuse.

Axoplasmic transport is an important physiologic function of the nerve cell. Amino acids taken up by the nerve cell bodies can be incorporated into proteins that can then be transported distally through the axon cylinders to reach the presynaptic terminals. This movement of proteins and substrates from the cytoplasm of the cell body through the cytoplasm of the axon is known as axoplasmic transport. The communication to and from the cell body

is therefore vitally important for the integrity of the nerve fiber.

The relation of the physiologic process of axoplasmic transport to mechanical low back pain is not immediately apparent until the site of the cell bodies of the dorsal root ganglion is recognized. Their location in the lumbosacral region in particular leaves them vulnerable to injury, which potentially compromises this important function. The vulnerability of the dorsal root ganglion is such that dorsal root ganglion injury potentially alters axoplasmic transport physiology, and thus interferes with dorsal nerve root function. Injured dorsal nerve roots in turn alter the type and quality of information that reaches the dorsal horn of the spinal cord.

What are these relations between cell body location, axoplasmic transport, and nerve root function that can be integrated into a discussion of mechanical low back pain? The axon cylinder, an extension of the cell body, de-

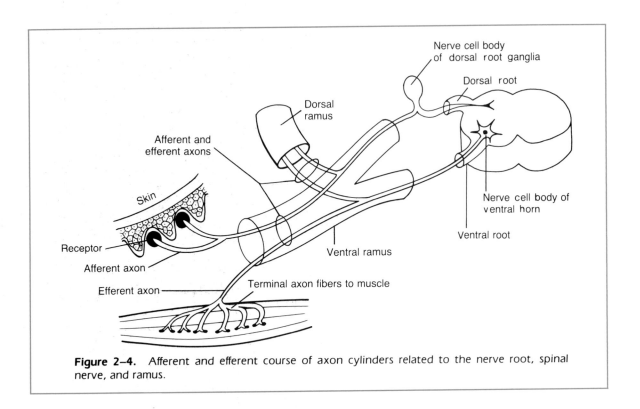

Figure 2–4. Afferent and efferent course of axon cylinders related to the nerve root, spinal nerve, and ramus.

pends on axoplasmic transport to ensure its proper function, since it utilizes the various proteins synthesized in the cell body for its synaptic activity. The nucleus of the nerve cell body is essential for the synthesis of proteins, which can then be carried by this axoplasmic flow to replace those proteins that have been degraded owing to nerve cell activity.

Because the cell body is so important for proper nerve cell function, the location of the dorsal root ganglion is of special importance in the lumbosacral region (see Fig. 2–3). Located in the intervertebral foramen or immediately subjacent to the pedicle of the vertebrae, the cell bodies of the dorsal root ganglion are easily subjected to mechanical stresses. As mentioned earlier, the unique nature of the dorsal root ganglion is such that each nerve cell body has two axon cylinders. One extends centrally to the spinal cord and the other, peripherally to the receptors located in the tissues. Altered axon (nerve fiber) function can occur as a result of injury to these nerve cell bodies because of interference with the axoplasmic transport process.[12]

The cell bodies that reside in the ventral horn of the spinal cord are equally as important, from the perspective of axoplasmic transport, as the cell bodies of the dorsal root ganglion; however, they are not located in as vulnerable a position. Nerve cell bodies, whether they be those of the dorsal root ganglion or those of the ventral horn cell, are important to the overall function of the axon cylinders that combine to form the nerve roots. Myelinated and unmyelinated axons extend from the cell bodies to form the dorsal roots and from the ventral horn cells to form the ventral roots.

The discussion above centered on injury to the cell body. If the nerve root itself is injured, then interference with its normal function, owing to interruption of axoplasmic transport, also results. Therefore, two mechanical causes can interfere with axoplasmic transport: damage to the axon cylinder (the nerve root itself) and injury to the cell bodies (dorsal root ganglion or anterior horn cell). Injury of either nerve root potentially alters the sensory or motor system.[28]

FORMATION OF THE NERVE ROOT SLEEVE

The nerve root, with its very thin covering of pia mater, invaginates the arachnoid and dura mater close to the intervertebral foramen (see Fig. 2–3). In this region the dural covering closely invests the nerve root in the form of a dural sleeve.

The nerve root, with its pial covering, must pierce the arachnoid and dura mater in the path from the spinal canal through the intervertebral foramen. The very thin arachnoid layer closely adheres to the inner surface of the dura. By adhering to the inner aspect of the dura in this way, a subarachnoid space is created around the nerve roots. The cerebrospinal fluid that bathes the nerve roots is contained in this space. The vasculature and cerebrospinal fluid are responsible for nourishing these nerve root structures, and are described later.

Bose and Balasubramaniam[6] have defined the anatomical pathway that the nerve root takes from the lateral aspect of the dural (thecal) sac to the intervertebral foramen as the nerve root canal. In this path from spinal canal to intervertebral foramen, the roots are anterior to the lamina, ligamentum flavum, and zygapophysial joint, and posterior to the intervertebral disc and vertebral body. The roots also lie immediately subjacent to the vertebral pedicle.

Narrowing of this nerve root canal owing to space-occupying lesions, such as spinal stenosis, hypertrophy of the ligamentous tissues in the spinal canal, and inflammatory conditions, can occur at its entrance, course, or exit. Any structure along the border of the nerve root canal can be involved. As noted by Hasue and coworkers[22] in their literature review and anatomical study of the lumbosacral nerve roots, the spatial relation between the nerve root and the osseus and nonosseus elements of the spinal canal and intervertebral foramen is clinically significant.

In the lumbar spinal canal the nerve roots float freely within the subarachnoid space of the thecal sac. Because of their mobility within this space, they can escape mechanical stresses. Therefore, compression of the lumbosacral nerve roots in the spinal canal is uncommon. However, as the roots exit laterally through the thecal tube, a funnel-shaped tube with a narrower diameter forms as the roots pick up a close investment of dura. This dural sleeve becomes attached to the nerve root close to the region of the intervertebral foramen. This fixation to the dura reduces the mobility of the roots and their ability to escape mechanical stresses. Therefore, the nerve roots become more vulnerable. This point is important in considering the convergence of forces that possibly result in nerve root irritation in the lumbopelvic region.

At the region of the intervertebral foramen the mobility of the dural sleeve itself is limited because the root sleeves may be anchored to the adjacent pedicle. Motion of the lumbar roots is, therefore, also limited.[45,52] Additionally, the anatomy of the intervertebral foramen and the tentlike shape of the dural sleeve preclude any excessive motion of the dura. The small excursion of the dural sleeve in an inferior and lateral direction, as might occur with a traction force to the root, effectively "plugs" the intervertebral foramen (Fig. 2–5).[55] This plugging of the intervertebral foramen by the dura mater is comparable to attempting to pull an A-frame tent through a doorway. The top of the tent can move a short distance through the doorway, but eventually the body of the tent plugs the doorway and prevents any further movement.

As noted by Louis,[33] the nerve root is dynamic, and elongation and changes in the direction of the roots of the cauda equina occur during movements. These movements result in traction forces to the nerve root and its dural sleeve. The unique method of dural investment and fixation helps to minimize the chance of nerve root avulsion from the spinal cord. However, this also leaves the nerve root with its dural sleeve more vulnerable to mechanical forces, since the limited mobility in the region of the intervertebral foramen does not allow easy escape from these forces.

Even though the dura mater is a tough fibrous tissue, the nerve roots are still considered more vulnerable than the peripheral nerves to potentially damaging insults such as

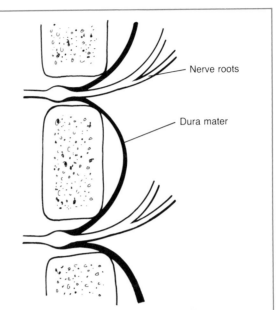

Figure 2–5. Protective function of the dura mater as it plugs the intervertebral foramen to minimize the potential for nerve root avulsion when a tensile force is imparted to the spinal nerve.

tensile and compression forces and to chemical irritation. The nerve roots lack the protective epineural and perineural coverings found in the peripheral nerves.[54,55] The connective tissue matrix of the epineurium and perineurium, with their fat cushions, offer the peripheral nerve a mechanism for protection against various mechanical stresses. The nerve root lacks this protection.

OSSEOUS AND NONOSSEOUS RELATIONS OF THE NERVE ROOTS AND DORSAL ROOT GANGLIA: IMPLICATIONS FOR ALTERED FUNCTION

The lumbosacral nerve roots, in their dural sleeves, are immediately adjacent to the osseous elements, and occupy a bony groove under the pedicle of the lumbar vertebrae commonly referred to as the lateral recess. It is in this subpedicular groove that the root sleeve, the ganglion associated with the dorsal root, and the nerve trunk lie along with branches of the lumbar arteries and veins, the lymphatics, and the sinu-vertebral nerve.[45] Immediately posterior to this complex is the ligamentum flavum, the anterior wall of the zygapophyseal joint capsule.

A close relation exists between the zygapophyseal joint with its anterior capsular contribution of the ligamentum flavum, and the nerve root and nerve root sleeve (Fig. 2–6). The wide variety of degenerative changes that are possible in the region of the zygapophyseal joint and ligamentum flavum, as well as the pedicle and intervertebral disc, can lead to the development of structural spinal stenosis. With stenotic conditions, additional mechanical stresses now reach the nerve root complex, and nerve root entrapment may result.

With the pathway that the nerve roots traverse more clearly defined, some detail of the dorsal root ganglion can now be added. As pre-

viously mentioned, the dorsal and ventral roots approach the intervertebral foramen within the dural sheath. The dorsal root joins the dorsal root ganglion, which is usually located in the approximate center of the intervertebral foramen.[48] Vanderlinden[56] has reported on a series of patients whose dorsal root ganglion was at the more medial aspect of the intervertebral foramen and within the nerve root canal itself in the subpedicular groove.

The dorsal root ganglion is composed of nerve cell bodies of various sizes.[30] Various neuropeptides are manufactured and reside in these cell bodies, although their physiologic roles have not been fully elucidated. The processes that extend from the nerve cell bodies travel in opposite directions. One process travels toward the spinal cord through the dorsal roots, and the other process travels toward the periphery through the spinal nerves.

At the terminal end of the peripheral processes (those processes destined for the peripheral tissues) are the various receptors of the joints and tissues, such as the articular mechanoreceptors, muscle spindles, Golgi tendon organs, and nociceptors (Fig. 2–7). Quite simply, the cell bodies for all sensory receptors are located together in the dorsal root ganglion, and they use the central process, which is the dorsal root, to convey their information into the central nervous system. Normal function is such that stimulation of the receptor initiates an action potential that travels along the peripheral process toward the cell body of the dorsal root ganglion. From the cell body the action potential travels along the dorsal nerve root and into the dorsal horn of the spinal cord.

The action potential traveling through the dorsal nerve root results in the release of neurotransmitters at the dorsal horn of the spinal cord that interact with synaptic endings of various neurons in the spinal cord. These neurotransmitters are peptides that are synthesized in the nerve cell bodies. The importance of axoplasmic transport is thus underscored, since this is one of the primary methods of moving the transmitter from the cell body to the synaptic ending of the axon.

Because pain is the most common complaint with disorders of the lumbopelvic region, one neuropeptide of interest is substance P. Sub-

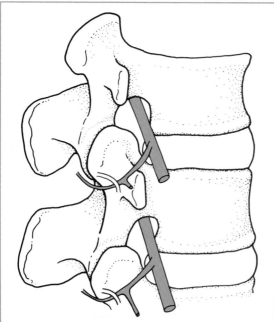

Figure 2–6. Relation of the zygapophyseal joint to the nerve root complex and the medial branch of the dorsal ramus.

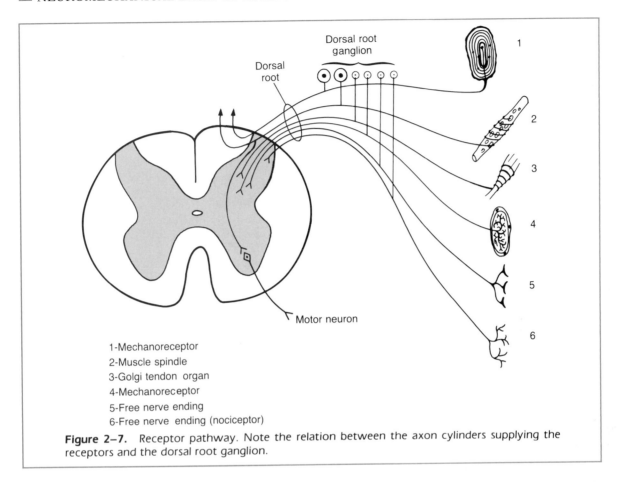

1-Mechanoreceptor
2-Muscle spindle
3-Golgi tendon organ
4-Mechanoreceptor
5-Free nerve ending
6-Free nerve ending (nociceptor)

Figure 2–7. Receptor pathway. Note the relation between the axon cylinders supplying the receptors and the dorsal root ganglion.

stance P (as well as other neuropeptides) is involved with processing sensory information that reaches the dorsal horn of the spinal cord through the dorsal nerve roots. This neuropeptide is a primary neurotransmitter of nociceptive afferent fibers that are thought to subserve the sensation of pain.[57] It is one of the neurotransmitters synthesized in the dorsal root ganglion, and is present in small nerve fibers of both the peripheral and central nervous systems.[13,15,58]

After being manufactured in the cell bodies of the dorsal root ganglion, substance P travels through the nerve fiber cylinders by axoplasmic transport to be distributed to the axon terminals. Recall that the axons leaving the cell bodies of the dorsal root ganglion travel both centrally (toward the spinal cord) and periph-

erally (toward the tissues). The release of substance P into the dorsal horn of the spinal cord results in synaptic activity of secondary neurons involved with the nociceptive pathways. The release of substance P into the tissues results in cutaneous vasodilation.[29]

Weinstein[58] and Badalamente and associates[1] have suggested that mechanical stimulation of the dorsal root ganglia increases production of substance P in the cell bodies, and increases the amount transported centrally to the substantia gelatinosa. The substantia gelatinosa is the region of the dorsal horn concerned with pain transmission. Through complex neurophysiology not fully understood, it appears that mechanical stimuli of the ganglia have the potential to initiate chemical changes in the cell bodies of the dorsal root ganglion.

The dorsal root ganglion is a mechanically sensitive structure in comparison to the nerve root. This is a major difference between compression of the normal nerve root and compression of the normal dorsal root ganglion. Compression of the normal dorsal root ganglion results in repetitive depolarization of the nerve cell bodies that constitute it.[25] Nerve cell activity results in the generation of action potentials. The increase in afferent activity to the spinal cord may initiate the neural pathways responsible for eliciting pain and also alter the sensorimotor reflex activity that contributes to the contractile state or resting tension of muscle.

The nerve root response to mechanical stresses is different from the dorsal root ganglion and is explored in the next section. In the lumbosacral region the space around the nerve root is widest in the spinal canal and narrowest in the intervertebral foramen.[22] As the nerve roots course through the spinal canal, the space is typically wide and unobstructed. As the roots approach the intervertebral foramen the exit narrows considerably. At the intervertebral foramen the nerve roots are supported and cushioned by the fat-containing connective tissue.[55] Transforamenal ligaments also bridge the opening of the intervertebral foramen.[3] Nevertheless, there is still ample room for the nerve root and its associated vasculature in the intervertebral foramen.

INJURED VERSUS NONINJURED NERVE ROOTS: THE UNIQUENESS OF NOURISHMENT MECHANISMS FOR LUMBOSACRAL NERVE ROOTS

The nerve root is subjected to many mechanical stresses throughout daily activities. For example, lumbar extension should, theoretically, place a compressive force on the nerve roots. Observation of a person performing the activities of daily living, however, reveals that a painful response does not occur every time the spine is extended. Likewise, the athlete's hamstring stretch clearly places a tensile force on the nerve root by way of the sciatic nerve, but it is essentially a pain-free activity.

Yet in some people with clear radicular problems, even the slightest extension movement of the lumbar spine appears to increase the compression on the nerve root, or a straight-leg raise of only 30 degrees appears to increase nerve root tension. The resulting painful response is disproportionate to the apparent force on the nerve root. Why are these nerve roots more responsive to mechanical stress, and what is the difference between normal and injured nerve roots?

The lumbosacral roots have some unique and clinically important characteristics that give insight to this question. Park and Watanabe[44] note that the lumbosacral nerve roots are structurally, vascularly, and metabolically unique regions of the nervous system. They are distinct structures when compared with the peripheral nerves. The neural fibers of the nerve roots are freestanding tracts, and they do not become incorporated into nerve bundles until they pierce the dural sheath.[44] Recall how the rootlets attach to the spinal cord and eventually form these nerve fiber bundles. A tight, compact nerve bundle structure does not begin to form until the root gets closer to the intervertebral foramen. The rootlets and freestanding fibers more closely resemble spinal cord tissue than peripheral nerve tissue. The nerve roots are not only functionally distinct, but also anatomically different from the peripheral nerves.

Because of this important difference, the vascular supply to the nerve roots more closely resembles the vascular supply to the central nervous system tissue than that to the peripheral nerve tissue. Vasculature to the lumbosacral roots relies on circulation stemming from the vascular plexus of the spinal cord. This vasculature follows the rootlets outward to partially nourish the nerve root.

The peripheral and central portions of the nerve roots, including the rootlets, also receive nourishment from a branching of the lumbar segmental arteries, which give rise to a microvascular system, plus the vessels of the spinal cord. This circulation, however, accounts for only 35 per cent of the nutritional source for the nerve root. This is a major physiologic difference between the nerve root and the peripheral nerve, which by comparison obtains 95 per cent of its nutrition from the vasculature.[44,49]

The nerve roots receive the remainder of their nutrition from the cerebrospinal fluid in which they are bathed. This is a significant contribution, and accounts for 58 per cent of nerve root nutrition owing to diffusion of the nutrients from the cerebrospinal fluid through the thin covering of pia mater and into the nerve root (totals less than 100 per cent because of experimental procedure; see ref. 49). In relying on diffusion as a method to allow nutrients into the nerve roots, it should be apparent that inflammatory conditions would impede this mechanism, and therefore adversely affect the nerve root. This factor is of fundamental importance in understanding the concepts of lumbosacral nerve root ischemia, nerve root irritation caused by an inflammatory process, and the biomechanics of the nerve root and associated vasculature.

With this basic understanding of the anatomy, nerve root pain mechanisms can be further developed. In experimental studies in which compressive forces were applied to noninjured nerve roots, MacNab[34] noted that the subjects experienced numbness and paresthesia but did not complain of pain. The healthy nerve root appears to be protected from eliciting a painful response when subjected to mechanical stresses. Even though the nerve root has close relations with many tissues in the path from the spinal canal to the intervertebral foramen, there appears to be a safeguard against continuous pain that may result from forces on the root.

Smyth and Wright,[51] however, studied nerve roots that were previously injured as a result of intervertebral disc lesions. In their experiments, pain did result from forces placed on the injured roots. The difference between these two experiments is that stress was placed on noninjured nerve roots in one instance and on injured nerve roots in another, with different experimental outcomes.

McCarron and coworkers[40] have shed further light on this aspect of injured nerve roots and, in particular, inflammation of the nerve roots. In their experiments with a homogenate of nucleus pulposus material, they were able to demonstrate that the nucleus pulposus acts as a chemical or an immunogenic irritant to the nerve root. The nerve roots and dural sac showed varying degrees of inflammatory response, ranging from edema and fibrin formation to increased vascularity and regional fibrosis, when exposed to this nucleus pulposus material. Inflammation or fibrosis of the root presents a physical impediment to the diffusion of nutrients from the cerebrospinal fluid through the membrane of the nerve root. This in turn leads to neuroischemic conditions that prevent or delay the delivery of essential nutrients normally supplied by the microvasculature.

An alteration in the nutritional status of the nerve root can result in minor damage to the axons. There is good evidence that axonal damage can cause mechanical sensitivity at the traumatized region and alter the spontaneous and evoked activity of the damaged axon segment and its dorsal root ganglion.[9,25,32]

Therefore, there is a strong suggestion that it is not the mechanical pressure alone that causes the phenomena of nerve root pain, but rather an abnormal chemical environment of the nerve root that alters electrical activity. The mechanical stresses lower the depolarization threshold, with resultant action potentials, which in turn initiate the nociceptive response.

In recalling the osseous and nonosseous elements that the nerve root must traverse, it should be apparent that an inflammatory response caused by injury of any of the tissues along the pathway has the potential to alter nerve root function by changing its nutritional status. Injury to any of these other tissues yields the same effect on the nerve root: altered nutritional status, an inflammatory response, and an irritated nerve root.

In summary, the major clinical considerations for involvement of the nerve root complex based on its structure and function include the following:

1. Inflammatory conditions of the nerve root complex

2. Fibrotic, scarred nerve roots with a resultant potential for decreased percolation of

nutrients from the cerebrospinal fluid of the subarachnoid space and into the nerve root

3. Neuroischemia of the root complex

4. Injury or mechanical irritation of the dorsal root ganglion

5. Relative immobility of the nerve root and sheath at the region of the nerve root canal that leaves it potentially vulnerable to abnormal forces.

CLINICAL ASPECTS: REFERRED PAIN VERSUS NERVE ROOT INVOLVEMENT

It is now well recognized that low back pain with concurrent lower extremity pain is not necessarily due to nerve root involvement. The results of experimental studies have shown that nearly all lumbopelvic tissues are capable of causing localized back pain as well as pain in the lower extremities. Irritation of the zygapophysial joint capsule, sacroiliac joint, dura mater, low back musculature, annulus fibrosus, and interspinous ligaments has been shown to give rise to symptoms in the lower extremities as well as in the low back.[17,27,31,39,42] Pain in the lower extremities owing to involvement of the lumbopelvic tissues or viscera is typically known as referred pain, whereas pain from the nerve root complex itself is known as radicular, or root, pain.

A satisfactory neuroanatomical pathway for the phenomenon of referred pain has not been described. Cyriax has given referred pain the simplest definition by calling it "pain felt elsewhere than at its true site."[14] Although this definition is adequate as a working clinical description, it only describes the phenomenon as perceived by the patient and observed by the clinician. Little is known about the definitive pathways and multitude of central nervous system synapses that are involved in referred pain.

The central nervous system, rather than the peripheral nervous system, is probably responsible for referred pain. As stated by Grieve, "pain happens within the central nervous system, and does not reside in the damaged local-

ity, though it may be perceived so."[21] By this is meant that the subjective experience of pain is the result of processing the afferent impulse at the spinal cord, brain stem, and cerebral cortex levels. The painful stimulus activates many pools of neurons within the central nervous system, some which result in the perception of referred pain.

Referred pain is well recognized and has given rise to the various dermatome, myotome, and sclerotome charts. These charts are used because embryologic segmentation is thought to be a predictor for patterns of referred pain. Although these charts may be helpful in some instances, segmental overlap is common, and it is still not possible to definitively determine the tissue of injury solely based on a distinct referred pain pattern.

In the strictest sense, pain from irritation of the nerve root or nerve root complex can also be considered referred pain because symptoms are felt at a distance from the source of irritation. The dura mater of the spinal canal, the nerve root sleeve, and the nerve root itself are pain-sensitive structures that are innervated by the sinuvertebral nerve (see below), and have the potential to refer pain to distal regions.

However, the clinician usually classifies pain in the lower extremities that results from involvement of the nerve root as radicular pain, and such pain that results from involvement of any other lumbopelvic tissue as referred pain. This distinction, although not anatomically correct, will be kept for the following discussion.

The nerve root can be clinically involved in two ways: *nerve root compression* and *nerve root irritation*. The clinical phenomenon of nerve root compression is most easily explained based on the current understanding of axon function. Compression of the axon cylinder alters its conduction capabilities. Consequently signs of nerve root dysfunction are expected when the nerve roots themselves are compressed. This compressive phenomenon can occur at any point along the pathway from the spinal canal to the intervertebral foramen.

A neurologic screen that examines sensory and motor root function should be included in all low back examinations. Table 2–1 lists sam-

TABLE 2–1. Neurologic Screening Examination for Nerve Root Compression

Test Type	Roots Evaluated
Reflexes	
Quadriceps	L3–L4
Tibialis posterior	L4–L5
Gastroc-soleus	S1–S2
Muscle	
Hip flexors	L2–L3
Quadriceps	L3–L4
Anterior tibialis	L4
Extensor hallucis longus	L5
Peroneals	S1–S2
Gastroc-soleus	S1–S2
Hamstrings	L4–L5
Gluteus maximus	L5–S1
Sensory	
Medial side of leg/foot	L4
Lateral side of leg/foot	L5
Posterior/posterolateral leg or thigh	S1–S2

ple tests for a nerve root screening examination that provide information about the integrity of the lumbosacral nerve roots and alert the clinician to possible neurologic involvement. Figure 2–8 shows patient positioning and sequencing that allow for an expeditious testing procedure.

These neurologic tests are designed to evaluate altered reflex activity, muscle weakness or wasting, and paresthesia and numbness in a clearly demarcated area. Because these tests are not used to evaluate pain, they tend to provide objective data, although a certain amount of subjectivity is inherent in any sensory test or request for motor activity.

Whereas nerve root compression results in changes in axon function that are, in many cases, measurable, nerve root irritation is not as clearly understood. Recall the discussion above pointing out that compression of the normal nerve root does not typically result in pain. However, the injured or irritated nerve root does give rise to pain when it is subjected to mechanical distortion. This increased sensitivity is the direct result of an inflammatory process to the nerve root. Extruded nuclear ma-terial from intervertebral disc degeneration, and irritation resulting from osseous entrapment of the root are two common causes that initiate an inflammatory response.

Morris and colleagues[43] helped to further distinguish between nerve root involvement owing to disc prolapse and nerve root involvement owing to bony entrapment. The results of their study showed that the most striking clinical effects of bony entrapment are the neurologic signs associated with nerve root involvement, whereas nerve root irritation signs (discussed below) are associated with the inflammatory changes produced by disc prolapse. If the nerve root is the site of a chronic inflammatory state, minor mechanical deformation has the potential to induce radiating pain.

With root irritation there is typically more lower extremity pain in a demarcated area than there is back pain. The areas of pain in the lower extremity follow dermatomal patterns more closely than other lumbopelvic tissues that refer pain into the lower extremity. Typically the patient complains more about the lower extremity pain than the low back pain, and the quality of the pain is usually sharper and more stabbing with nerve root irritation. Because the roots most commonly involved are the last two lumbar and the first sacral, the complaints of lower extremity pain are usually focused in the leg.

Different mechanical stresses can be placed on the irritated nerve root and its accompanying investments. Maitland[35] describes the "slump test," which maximally stresses the dural sheath and the nerve roots (Fig. 2–9). This test exerts a cephalad and caudally directed force on the dura mater, and additionally places a tensile stress on the nerve roots of the lower extremity.[35] From the sitting position, the patient slumps forward, which flexes the thoracic and lumbar spine. Overpressure is applied through the shoulders to increase the flexion force. Head and neck flexion are then added to the position. While the patient maintains this position, the knee is extended and the ankle dorsiflexed.

The test is instructive in the mechanics of the nerve roots and their coverings within the spinal canal and intervertebral foramen. The

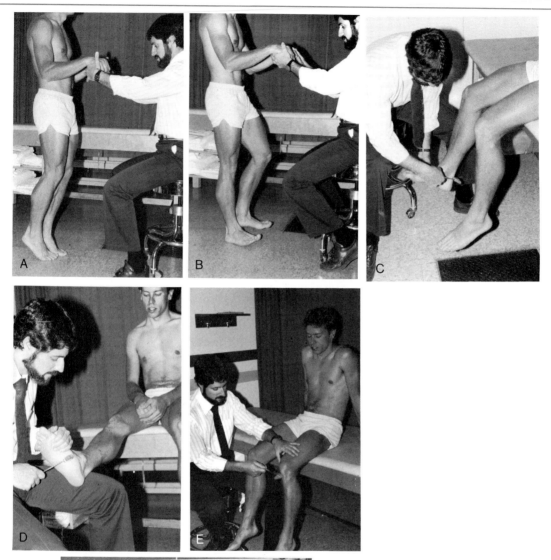

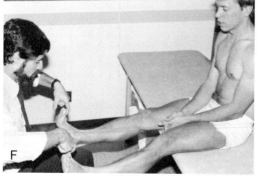

Figure 2–8. Neurological screening examination. The exam is provided in a standing, sitting, supine lying and prone lying sequence to minimize position changes by the patient. *A*, Toe walking. Examiner detects patient pushing down on supporting hands. *B*, Heel walking. *C*, Gastroc-soleus reflex. *D*, Posterior tibialis reflex. *E*, Quadriceps reflex. *F*, Extensor hallucis longus muscle test.

Illustration continued on opposite page.

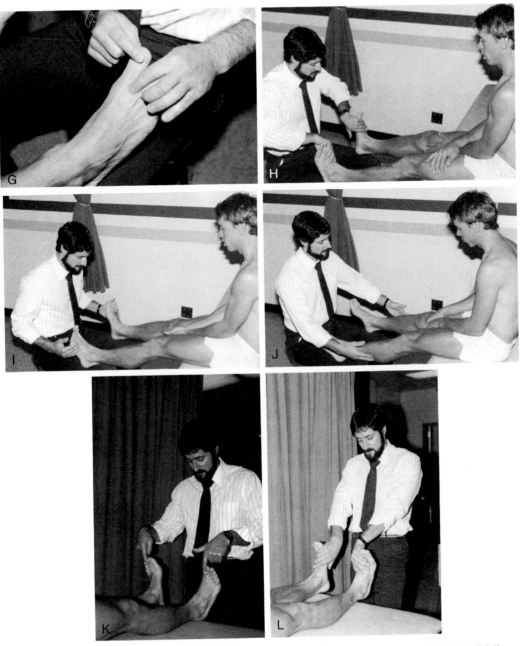

Figure 2–8 *Continued   G,* Examiner contact for extensor hallucis longus test. *H,* Anterior tibialis muscle test. *I,* Peroneal muscle test. *J,* Sensory exam. *K,* Supine extensor hallucis longus test. Rechecking in supine helps substantiate previous findings of the neurological screen. *L,* Supine anterior tibialis test.

Illustration continued on following page.

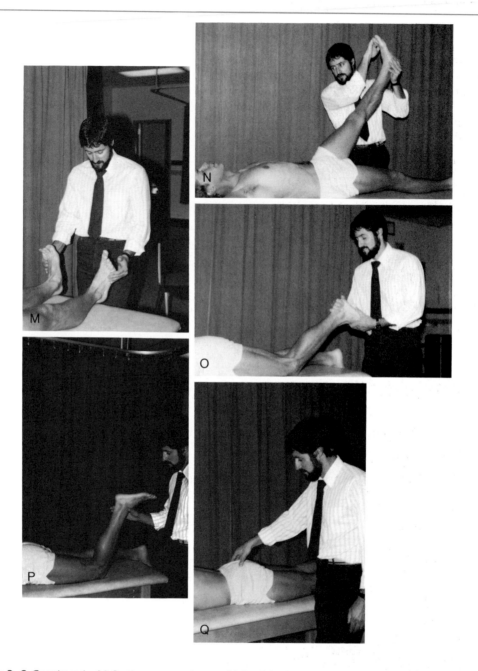

Figure 2–8 *Continued*   *M*, Supine peroneals test. *N*, Straight leg raise. *O*, Hamstring muscle test. *P*, Quadriceps muscle test. *Q*, Palpation for "setting" the gluteus maximus.

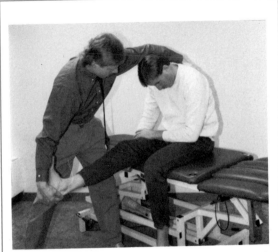

Figure 2–9. Slump test as described by Maitland.

minutes of injecting local anesthetic into the zygapophyseal joint spaces. It would thus seem logical to conclude that a limitation of straight-leg raising can also occur because of zygapophyseal joint involvement.

Why would irritation of another lumbopelvic tissue such as the zygapophyseal joint show a limitation in straight-leg raising? A plausible explanation takes into account the reflex nature of afferent and efferent information. When any structure of the lumbopelvic region or viscera is injured and initiates the volley of impulses into the dorsal horn of the spinal cord, altered efferent motor patterns can occur as a result of reflex activity at the central nervous system level. This increase in efferent output to the muscles of the lower extremities, such as the hamstrings and other hip extensors, may limit the motion that occurs in the straight-leg raise, but such results should not be classified as positive. This is one reason both the increase and the location of the pain in the lower ex-

examiner now has the ability to decrease or increase the tension on the dura or nerve roots by varying the degree of neck flexion or knee extension, or any other component of the final position. The relation between the pain response of the patient and the varying amounts of tension can then be used to assess the degree and severity of nerve root irritation.[35]

One of the most common tests used is the straight-leg raise test. With nerve root irritation leg pain may be exacerbated as the lower extremity is raised. By incorporating internal rotation and adduction of the hip during the straight-leg raise test, an even greater tensile force is placed on the nerve roots by way of the sciatic nerve.[7] This increased tensile force placed on the nerve root is due to the course that the sciatic nerve takes as it travels lateral to the ischial tuberosity (Fig. 2–10). This bony protuberance acts as a fulcrum during the maneuver. Other methods to increase the tensile force on the nerve root include ankle dorsiflexion and manual compression by the examiner in the popliteal fossa.

Mooney and Robertson,[42] in their classic study of the zygapophyseal joints, showed that reduced straight-leg raising as a result of lumbar joint injection could be improved within

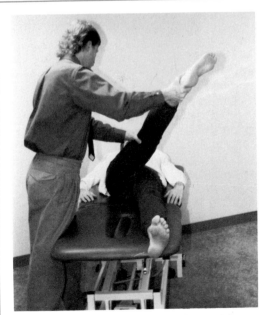

Figure 2–10. Adding hip adduction and internal rotation to the straight-leg raise test increases the tensile stress to the lumbosacral nerve roots.

tremity, rather than the simple limitation of range of motion, should be closely scrutinized during the straight-leg raise. If a nerve root is injured, the increased tension on the irritated nerve roots should be a sufficient mechanical stimulus to intensify the pain along the root distribution in the lower extremity.

When the clinician assesses the result of any test that evaluates range of motion, such as the straight-leg raise test or a test for hip hyperextension capabilities, he should determine whether the limitation of motion is due to increased efferent output from the central nervous system to the muscles, resulting in an increase in their stiffness, or to adaptive shortening. Oftentimes the reflex motor activity is in response to an injured nerve root or because of protective muscle guarding. Although adaptively shortened tissues may need to be stretched, the muscles should be carefully assessed to determine if stretching is indicated.

The results of Mooney and Robertson's study also showed that depressed reflexes were restored after injection of anesthetic into the apophyseal joints.[42] This helps to underscore the fact that a painful structure, such as a joint, that is initiating nociceptive activity (afferent volley of action potentials to the dorsal horn) into the spinal cord has the potential to reflexly alter efferent motor activity (connections with the ventral horn cells).

It should not be construed that synaptic events at the level of the spinal cord are the only central nervous system activities that are occurring. It is probable that other regions of the spinal cord, as well as the brain stem and the cerebral cortex, are involved in this complex circuitry. The important point is that increases or decreases of the painful stimulus change the afferent information reaching the dorsal horn of the spinal cord, which in turn alters central nervous system efferent activity.

Caution must be taken in interpreting tests for the nerve root, whether they be the motor, sensory, reflex, or straight-leg raise tests. By themselves they offer little in the way of diagnosis. However, as a group or combined with the history and other portions of the objective examination, the test results provide useful information.

INNERVATION OF LUMBOPELVIC TISSUES

In the spinal canal, motor and sensory information for human behavior is carried by individual nerve roots. These roots merge to form the spinal nerve, which is a very short segment. From the spinal nerve outward the motor and sensory components intertwine, and travel together by way of the ventral and dorsal primary rami (see Fig. 2–4). Therefore, although the dorsal and ventral roots are largely involved with sensory and motor information, respectively, the dorsal and ventral rami both carry motor and sensory information. It is these rami that then give rise to peripheral nerves, which continue on to innervate the lumbopelvic tissues.

On exiting the intervertebral foramen the spinal nerve immediately branches into the dorsal and ventral rami. The ventral rami pierce the psoas major muscle and merge with other ventral rami to form the lumbosacral plexus. Some of the branches of the ventral rami directly innervate the psoas major, psoas minor, and quadratus lumborum muscles, while others give rise to the numerous peripheral nerves that innervate the lower extremity. Cutaneous nerves to the anterior and medial thigh are also derived from the lumbosacral plexus or branch from the peripheral nerves of the thigh. Figure 2–11 shows the lumbosacral plexus with its motor and sensory branches.

The ventral rami are of great importance in understanding the motor and sensory innervation of the lower extremity. However, the dorsal rami and their branches assume great importance with regard to the innervation of the various lumbopelvic tissues. They are responsible for nearly all of the innervation of the posterior elements of the lumbopelvic region, which is an important point in considering low back pain. It is an accepted fact that in order to have pain after tissue injury, the tissues must be innervated. Therefore, it behooves us to completely understand the innervation of the lumbopelvic region, since low back pain is the most common musculoskeletal complaint seen in the clinical practice.

The dorsal ramus branches from the spinal

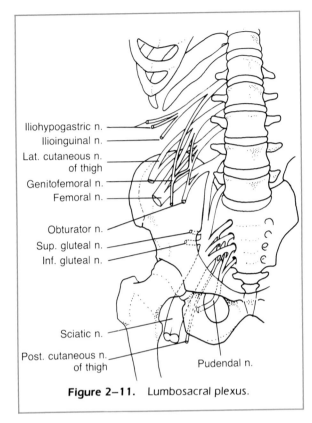

Iliohypogastric n.
Ilioinguinal n.
Lat. cutaneous n.
  of thigh
Genitofemoral n.
Femoral n.

Obturator n.
Sup. gluteal n.
Inf. gluteal n.

Sciatic n.

Post. cutaneous n.
  of thigh   Pudendal n.

Figure 2–11. Lumbosacral plexus.

cussion, only the lateral and medial branches are considered.

The medial branch innervates the lumbopelvic tissues that are medial and adjacent to a parasagittal plane through the zygapophyseal joints (Fig. 2–12). Tissues that occupy the area between the spinous processes and the longitudinal plane of the zygapophyseal joints include the multifidus, rotatores, interspinalis, and intertransversarii musculature; the apophyseal joint structures; and the interspinous ligaments; they are, therefore, innervated by the medial branch of the dorsal rami.

Tissues that are lateral to the apophyseal joint plane are innervated by the lateral branches of the dorsal rami. They include the iliocostalis and longissimus muscles of the erector spinae and the thoracolumbar fascia.[4] However, Ikari[26] was unable to trace free nerve endings in the most superficial layer of thoracolumbar fascia.

The lateral branches of the dorsal rami of L1, L2, and L3 eventually become cutaneous in

nerve, turns posteriorly, and then courses through the tissues of the lumbopelvic region. The L5 dorsal ramus is longer and has a more tortuous course than the other dorsal rami as it follows the alar and dorsal surfaces of the sacrum.[5] Both the afferent information coming from the lumbopelvic tissues to the central nervous system and the efferent information coming from the central nervous system to the muscles of the lumbopelvic region must traverse the dorsal rami or the previously mentioned ventral rami.

Figure 2–12 shows the path of the dorsal rami and their associated branches. The two largest branches are the medial and lateral divisions. Bogduk and associates[5] note that careful dissection of these medial and lateral branches of the dorsal rami can reveal a third branch, the intermediate branch. This branch appears to be an intermediate branch of the lateral ramus, but for the purposes of this dis-

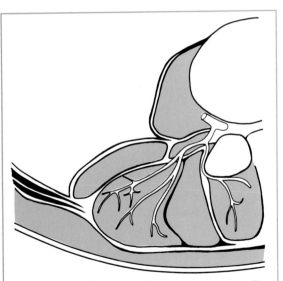

Figure 2–12. The path of the dorsal ramus. The medial branch of the dorsal ramus courses under the zygapophyseal joint, while the lateral branch courses through the erector spinae muscle. (Adapted from The Neurobiologic Mechanisms of Manipulative Therapy, ed. Irvin M. Korr. Plenum Press, New York, 1978.)

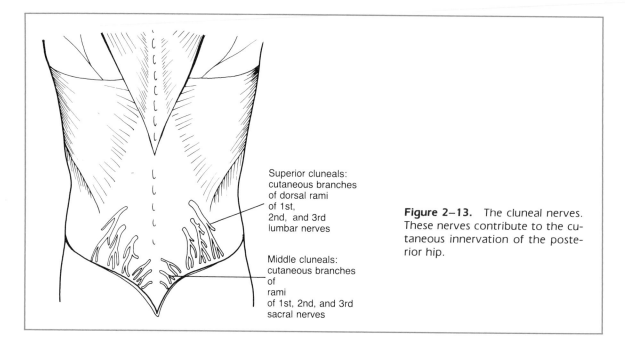

Superior cluneals:
cutaneous branches
of dorsal rami
of 1st,
2nd, and 3rd
lumbar nerves

Figure 2–13. *The cluneal nerves. These nerves contribute to the cutaneous innervation of the posterior hip.*

Middle cluneals:
cutaneous branches
of
rami
of 1st, 2nd, and 3rd
sacral nerves

their course through the iliocostalis and longissimus muscles to supply the skin. Hollinshead and Rosse[24] refer to these upper three lumbar nerves as the superior cluneal nerves. They pierce the superficial fascia above the iliac crest and descend to supply the skin over the buttock. The middle cluneal nerves are the lateral branches of the dorsal rami of the first three sacral nerves; they extend more laterally to innervate skin toward the region of the greater trochanter (Fig. 2–13).

This description of tissues innervated by the medial and lateral branches of the dorsal rami indicates that both sensory and motor innervation are provided by these nerves. The motor innervation to the skeletal muscles of the lumbopelvic region, and the nociceptive, proprioceptive, and kinesthetic sensory qualities from the joint structures, osseous elements, and soft tissues of the low back are carried by these divisions. An understanding of this innervation is important in order to appreciate the anatomical pathways that are used for sensory feedback and muscle activity and that contribute to motor control. This is further discussed in the next section.

The final important component of lumbopelvic tissue innervation is the sinuvertebral nerves. These nerves innervate structures within the spinal canal. Also known as the recurrent nerves, they are branches of the spinal nerve or ventral rami that are joined by branches from the grey ramus communicans of the sympathetic chain. The nerve then traverses a path back into the intervertebral foramen (Fig. 2–14).

Structures within the spinal canal, such as the ventral aspect of the dura mater, epidural vasculature, posterior longitudinal ligament, posterior aspect of the annulus fibrosus, and basivertebral veins as they enter the vertebral body, are innervated by the sinuvertebral nerve.[4] Because these nerves do not innervate skeletal muscle structures, their fibers are probably afferent, carry sensory qualities such as nociception and proprioceptive feedback to the central nervous system and are efferent to the smooth muscle of the vasculature. In addition to its visceral motor function, the sinuvertebral nerve may simply utilize the gray ramus as a path toward its final destination.[3]

The innervation of the intervertebral disc

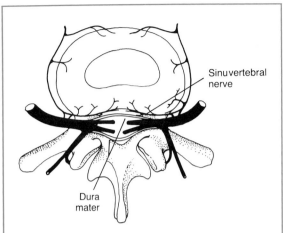

Figure 2–14. The sinuvertebral nerve. This nerve courses back through the intervertebral foramen to innervate structures within the spinal canal.

deserves special mention. Although most authorities agree that the nucleus pulposus is not innervated, the annulus fibrosus, especially its outer aspect, appears to be innervated. Malinsky[36] not only described nerve fibers ramifying in the outer rings of the annulus, but also the various types of nerve endings in the outer annulus and on its surface. He also noted that these receptors were more abundant in the lateral regions of the disc.

This study must also be correlated with Bogduk's[4] dissections. Bogduk notes that the posterolateral aspect of the disc is innervated by the ventral and grey rami, the lateral aspect by the ascending and descending branches of the grey rami, and the anterior aspect (including the anterior longitudinal ligament) by branches from the sympathetic plexus adjacent to the vertebral body. The remaining posterior aspect of the annulus fibrosus and the posterior longitudinal ligament are innervated by the sinuvertebral nerve.

These peripheral nerve fibers described by Bogduk[4] terminate in the intervertebral disc as free nerve endings, and are associated with nonencapsulated receptors, as described by Malinsky.[36] Yoshizawa and coworkers[60] also confirmed the presence of nerve fibers, free

nerve endings, and various types of receptors in the intervertebral disc.

Because nerve fibers with their free nerve endings and receptors have been found within the annulus, it is tempting to speculate as to their function. Certainly pain from mechanical or chemical irritation of the free nerve endings appears reasonable, and thus annular injury may result in primary discogenic pain. Primary discogenic pain typically has broad, ill-defined boundaries.[23] With discogenic pain the patient usually describes a broad, nonspecific band across the back or gluteal region. The pain may spread into the upper posterior or posterolateral thigh and across the abdomen.[35] Maitland[35] describes the quality of pain as "distressing, wearing, sickening and depressing." This is a different painful quality than the aching and discomfort from injured ligamentous structures.

The innervation of the disc and the receptor system involved also lead to speculation about a proprioceptive function of the intervertebral disc. Certainly the various compression, torsion, and tensile forces to the annulus have the potential to stimulate these receptors in a variety of spatial and temporal patterns. Although conclusive evidence of the function of the disc is still missing, Farfan[16] points out that it is tempting to conceive of the disc as being the largest sense organ in the body that influences postural mechanisms. This idea is based on the premise that afferent neurologic information produced by forces on the disc result in reflex connections with neurons involved in the motor pathways. Motor activity is modified, and results in postural changes and adaptations to the various forces placed on the spine.

THE RECEPTOR SYSTEM: THE IMPORTANCE OF PROPRIOCEPTIVE AND KINESTHETIC INFORMATION

From a practical standpoint, it is helpful to divide neural function into two components: the sensory, or afferent, information that reaches the central nervous system from the tissues themselves and the motor, or efferent, information that leaves the central nervous system to innervate the effectors. Connections between these two systems are universally accepted; however, the detailed nature of the synapses and pathways through the spinal cord, brain stem, and cerebral cortex has not yet been fully elucidated. This section primarily focuses on the receptor system and its influence on motor behavior.

The components of the afferent system can be subdivided into the receptors that are located within the tissues and the peripheral sensory nerves that carry information toward the spinal cord. For the purpose of discussing the receptor system in relation to lumbopelvic function and dysfunction, the receptors can be further subdivided into (a) the nociceptive receptors, (b) skin and articular (joint) mechanoreceptors, and (c) receptors in the muscle and muscle-tendon units (muscle spindles and Golgi tendon organs).

Using the lumbopelvic tissues as an exam-ple, a centripetal pathway from the tissue receptor to the spinal cord can be detailed. The receptors, when activated by an appropriate stimulus of adequate magnitude, initiate an action potential that progresses through the nerve fibers of the medial or lateral division of the dorsal rami, the dorsal ramus itself, the spinal nerve, the dorsal root, and finally into the dorsal horn of the spinal cord.

Three examples of this centripetal flow of information from the tissues to the spinal cord are shown in Figure 2–15. These three pathways describe the common route used by the nociceptors, the articular mechanoreceptors, and the muscle spindles. Even though the sensory modality is different in each case, the afferent pathway to the dorsal horn of the spinal cord is similar. In the spinal cord the individual sensory modality is sorted into different tracts that influence other spinal cord levels as well as the brain stem, cerebellum, basal nuclei, and cerebral cortex.

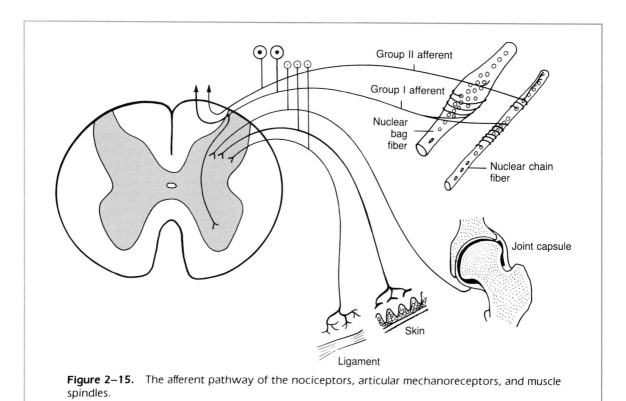

Figure 2–15. The afferent pathway of the nociceptors, articular mechanoreceptors, and muscle spindles.

THE NOCICEPTIVE RECEPTOR SYSTEM AND ITS ROLE IN THE ASSESSMENT OF LOW BACK PAIN

The nociceptive receptors are the least morphologically differentiated of the various types of receptors. They range from free nerve endings to plexiform arrangements of nerve fibers that ramify throughout the tissues.[59] Nociceptive receptors can be activated in three ways: mechanical pressure of sufficient severity, extreme heat, and chemical irritation. In dealing with the problem of low back pain, activation by excessive mechanical forces (although it is still not known whether the nociceptors respond directly to the noxious stimulus or indirectly by means of one or more chemical intermediaries released from the traumatized tissue) and chemical irritation are the most common causes.[37]

Theoretically, any innervated tissue of the lumbopelvic region is a potential source of pain. Although the disc has historically played a major role as a mediator of low back pain, nearly every other structure in the low back has also been shown to be a potential source of pain. With so many different structures being a nociceptive source, it is nearly impossible to isolate the one tissue at fault during a low back evaluation. Indeed, with an understanding of the anatomy and mechanics of spinal function, and recognition of the interplay of the various tissues, the chances of an isolated, single tissue being injured are remote.

The key to understanding the importance of the nociceptive response, however, lies in the clinician's ability to provoke familiar symptoms by imparting the *forces* that reproduce the nociceptive stimulus causing the patient's pain. The evaluation should be designed to identify the abnormal forces that stimulate a nociceptor and give rise to familiar pain. Treatment is then designed around the concept of minimizing this potentially destructive force.

At first glance this appears overly simplistic and a radical departure from the tissue identification methods of dealing with mechanical low back pain. The results of the Quebec Task Force on Spinal Disorders (1987), however, suggest that trying to diagnosis the tissue at fault is inadequate:

The literature is therefore replete with diagnostic terms: lumbar sprain, lumbar strain, lumbago, sciatica, discal hernia, discopathy, facet syndrome, lumbar myositis, ligamentitis, minor intervertebral displacement, dysfunction of the intervertebral joint, fibromyositis, fascitis, myofascitis, articular hypomobility and hypermobility, discarthrosis, metameric cellulotenoperiostomyalgic syndrome, posterior branch syndrome, rhizopathy, etc. Frequently, one finds in a patient's medical chart two or three of these diagnoses, made by different physicians, depending on whether they focused on the main symptom (acute lumbago), on the radiologic aspect (discarthrosis), or on a physiopathologic hypothesis (facet syndrome, minor intervertebral displacement, myofascitis, or disc degeneration). . . .

We therefore thought it necessary to propose an original classification that is not based solely on pathologic entities, since they remain too vague in most cases, but that reflects the clinical entities encountered in practice.[46]

When the myriad of sacroiliac diagnoses is added to the list above, we can certainly appreciate how the same mechanical low back pain syndrome ultimately results in numerous diagnoses that usually depend on clinician biases. Instead of focusing on the *forces* that activate the nociceptive receptors during evaluation, we have emphasized physiopathologic hypothesis and have used these hypotheses to rationalize the tissue we believe to be at fault. Treatment programs are then based on these biases. Unfortunately this disregards the normal synergistic behavior of all lumbopelvic tissues working together (and probably getting injured together), as well as current knowledge of neuroanatomy and neurophysiology.

Stimulation of nociceptors ultimately results in synaptic activity in the central nervous system. It is beyond the scope of this text to describe the centripetal flow of nociceptive information in order to give rise to the conscious appreciation of pain; these pathways are detailed in texts of neuroanatomy. However, the influence of the nociceptive stimulus on muscle activity should be recognized. The afferent sensory information from injured tissue alters efferent motor output primarily at a reflex level. This is not an undesirable situation in all instances. Assuming that altered motor activity occurs in order to minimize any chance of further injury or to adapt to the change in tissue status, then this neural activity can be a normal biologic function necessary for survival.

It should also be understood that there is a nociceptive threshold that probably correlates with the amount of tissue swelling. As the swelling decreases, the painful stimulus also decreases. The patient and clinician should recognize that although the pain might be decreased, complete healing has not necessarily occurred. If this feature is not recognized, it can predispose the person to reinjury.

THE MECHANORECEPTOR SYSTEM AND ITS ROLE IN MOTOR CONTROL

Mechanical low back pain can develop as a result of an abnormal movement pattern that loads the tissue at levels that exceed tissue tolerance. After injury a movement pattern may continually stress the lumbopelvic tissues above their tolerance. Changes in movement patterns become critical when tissue is injured because these changes have the potential to increase or decrease the destructive forces on injured tissue. In this regard, focusing on mechanical low back pain as a movement disorder appropriately changes the emphasis of evaluation and treatment.

Both reflex and conscious control of movement patterns occur because the articular mechanoreceptors, muscle spindles, and Golgi tendon organs convey sensory information to the central nervous system. These receptors play a unique role in influencing motor output because they provide proprioceptive and kinesthetic information. This information becomes the basis for motor control when it is processed at the various levels of the central nervous system. It is important for the clinician managing mechanical low back pain to be aware of the relation between these receptors and motor output because it is the scientific foundation for the various exercise, training, ergonomic, and back education programs used in the management of this problem.

Mechanoreceptors are biologic transducers that take a mechanical stimulus and convert it into electrical energy. This electrical energy initiates central nervous system responses. The multiple types of skin and joint receptors work together in both temporal and spatial summation patterns and inform the central nervous system of joint activity.[47]

The muscle spindles and Golgi tendon organs are also mechanoreceptors that provide important sensory information to the central nervous system. Because of their anatomical location, these receptors can convey information regarding the changing status of muscle activity. They play a major role in the conscious appreciation of proprioception and kinesthesia. For example, it has been found that we estimate joint angle from information about muscle length provided by the muscle spindle receptors.[37]

It is important to note the distinction between sensory information delivered to the central nervous system that does not reach consciousness and sensory information that reaches conscious awareness, since they are entirely different concepts. Not all sensory information reaches the conscious appreciation levels. Even though the articular receptors described previously deliver their information to the central nervous system, they are not the only contributors to the conscious aspects of proprioception and kinesthesia. Conscious awareness is also in part a result of muscle spindle activity with contribution by the articular receptors.[18,19,38] However, since many of our motor programs occur and are influenced by central nervous system activity at the subcortical level, afferent activity from all receptor sources is important because of their influence on the various motor centers in the spinal cord and brain.

The muscle spindles do not directly contribute to overall muscle tension; however, they indirectly play a major role. Because the spindle has contractile properties, it can shorten when stimulated by the gamma motor neuron. This contraction distorts the spindle, which subsequently results in afferent discharge to the central nervous system. The sophistication of the muscle spindle system is such that the two types of spindle fibers (bag and chain) differ in the types of contraction they can exhibit: slow contractions of the spindle are produced by the bag fibers, and fast contractions are produced by the chain fibers.[11] By having a variation of spindle contractions, distortion of the receptor portion of the spindle occurs at different rates and provides a variety of unique afferent information regarding the status of the muscle to the central nervous system.

Because the muscle spindle is arranged in parallel with the muscle fiber, it increases its rate of discharge whenever the muscle is stretched. The different types of spindle receptor allow it to be responsive to changes in the length of muscle as well as to the rate at which the changes in length occur. When the alpha motor neuron causes the extrafusal muscle fibers to contract, the tension on the muscle spindle activity tends to decrease because it is being "unloaded." However, because there is coactivation of the alpha and gamma motor neurons, the spindle, which is also contracting owing to gamma motor neuron firing, maintains some degree of tension rather than becoming completely "unloaded."

The Golgi tendon organs are connective tissue capsules that are located at the musculotendinous junction. Approximately 15 to 20 skeletal muscle fibers enter the capsule. The Golgi tendon organ is thus oriented in series with the muscle. Because of this anatomical arrangement, the Golgi tendon organ is activated by stretching the muscle, contracting the muscle, or both. The afferent nerve of the Golgi tendon organ enters the capsule and branches many times. As the muscle contracts or stretches, the collagen framework of the Golgi tendon organ becomes distorted. This distortion causes the axons to fire, and a flow of afferent information toward the central nervous system begins.

The Golgi tendon organ has a high threshold when activated by passive stretch. It was originally believed that the role of the Golgi tendon organ was protective, in that it prevented the muscle from producing excessive tension by inhibiting the motor neurons innervating the homonymous and synergistic muscles. It is now recognized that these receptors are extremely sensitive to muscle contraction and provide important feedback to the central nervous system, differentiating the degree of muscle tension during contraction. Because they are located at the musculotendinous junction

and are related to 15 to 20 extrafusal muscle fibers, it is conceivable that the force produced by just one motor unit can be recorded by these receptors.[8] Therefore, the Golgi tendon organ responds not only to the degree of stretch placed on the tendon, but also to any contraction by the muscle. As the muscle contracts, various gradations of force are used, depending on the desired results. These various gradations are sensed by the Golgi tendon organ, which in turn informs the central nervous system. A feedback loop evolves in which motor control is adjusted at the spinal cord, brain stem, and cerebral cortex levels.

The Golgi tendon organ, like the muscle spindle, also delivers afferent information to the cerebellum and assists in the regulation of motor output. The cerebellum is known to exert influence over the spinal cord, various nuclei of the brain stem that give rise to motor tracts, and the cerebral cortex, from which originates the corticospinal tracts.

The receptor system has been briefly described in order to provide a more comprehensive understanding of its influence on motor behavior. Consideration needs to be given to how the receptor system and muscles work as a unit. It is interesting to note, for example, that the pools of alpha motor neurons that innervate the skeletal muscle are in the same immediate location in the spinal cord as the gamma motor neurons that innervate the muscle spindle. Both pools are thus under direct influence of central motor tracts and the multiplicity of sensory stimuli that arise from the tissues. Smooth movement requires an integration of and balance between the afferent and the efferent aspects of motor behavior.

Afferent information is especially important in the timing and shaping of motor patterns. In the treatment of low back disorders there is need to include proprioceptive and kinesthetic awareness training of spinal positions and movements, especially those postures that have the potential to stimulate the nociceptive receptors in injured tissues.

In order to allow the patient to successfully manage his low back problem, it is necessary that he recognize the vulnerable positions of his lumbopelvic region that allow destructive forces to occur. The first step in restoring function in the rehabilitation process is teaching the patient what a vulnerable position for his particular spinal problem might be. These vulnerable and invulnerable positions are determined by the clinician during the evaluation process (see Chapter 5). The patient needs to develop proprioceptive awareness as to which positions are vulnerable and which invulnerable for his particular injury. Subsequent strengthening exercises are futile without recognition of this proprioceptive sense because the patient will probably continually invite reinjury. Training in this manner recognizes the importance of the afferent input reaching the central nervous system.

As a muscle is trained, changes in its resting tension can be seen. Although these changes are partly due to a remodeling of the muscle, a certain degree of central nervous system activation also occurs. Carew and Ghez[11] have compared the tension of the muscle with that of a spring. With a thicker spring, the stiffness increases (see Chapter 3). The stiffness of the muscle can also be increased by increasing the neural outflow to it. Recall that this neural outflow affects the gamma as well as the alpha motor systems. The gamma system plays a large part in biasing the spindle toward an increased sensitivity to movement. This increased potential for awareness of movement by the sensory receptors is in part a "training" mechanism in itself.

The central nervous system also makes important changes with proper exercise programs. This training is the result of an enhanced balance between the afferent sensory and efferent motor systems. Sensitivity toward movement is an important component of proprioceptive and kinesthetic strength training. Diminished proprioceptive feedback is characteristic of sedentary living and results in a reduction of the sensitivity of the spindle secondary afferents in antigravity muscles.[20] Recognition of this is probably the unifying element behind the myriad of back education programs now available. These programs teach the patient awareness of spine postures (proprioceptive awareness) and ultimately require a significant degree of muscle activity (muscle training).

Because all patients do not have similarly injured tissues, and the nociceptive response is variable owing to the different degree of mechanical or chemical irritation of the nociceptors, standardized treatment programs have little to offer the patient in the way of self-management. Consideration must be given to the importance of the afferent neurology of the region rather than simply teaching every patient to maintain one particular spine position or exercise one muscle group. Management in this manner ignores basic neurophysiology; that is, the person moves in a motor pattern appropriate for his strength, coordination, and connective tissue makeup. In many cases the low back pain patient has a movement pattern that perpetuates the nociceptive response. Recognition of this balance between afferent and efferent neurobiology is essential to understanding the function of the lumbopelvic region.

SUMMARY

The purpose of this chapter was to familiarize the clinician with selected aspects of neuroanatomy and neurophysiology of the lumbopelvic region. In particular, functional considerations were presented in a manner to stimulate the clinician to fully consider the importance of afferent neurobiology in the evaluation and treatment of lumbopelvic disorders.

Neuromechanical elements of lumbopelvic problems especially underscore the scientific foundations of pain and function. The treatment approach to dealing with low back pain, supported by the scientific literature, is rapidly changing to a focus on function in order to alter the disability.[10] As in rehabilitation of the extremities, optimal function is not simply "efferent" in nature—that is, absolute strength, or a significant aerobic capacity—but includes such factors as coordination, balance, and motor learning. This recognizes the important influence of the nervous system for optimal function. An early and safe return to activity after injury is just as important in maintaining central nervous system "health" as it is in maintaining musculoskeletal health. We suggest that restoration of function include an integration of the neuromusculoskeletal systems.

REFERENCES

1. Badalamente MA, Dee R, Ghillani R, et al: Mechanical stimulation of dorsal root ganglia induces increased production of substance P: A mechanism for pain following nerve root compromise? Spine-12:552, 1987.
2. Barr M: The Human Nervous System. Philadelphia, JB Lippincott, 1988.
3. Bogduk N: Clinical Anatomy of the Lumbar Spine. New York, Churchill Livingstone, 1987.
4. Bogduk N: The innervation of the lumbar spine. Spine 8:286, 1983.
5. Bogduk N, Wilson AS, Tynan W: The human lumbar dorsal rami. J Anat 134:383, 1982.
6. Bose K, Balasubramaniam P: Nerve root canals of the lumbar spine. Spine 9:16, 1984.
7. Breig A, Troup JDG: Biomechanical considerations in the straight leg raising test. Spine 4:243, 1974.
8. Brodal A: Neurological Anatomy Related to Clinical Medicine. Oxford, Oxford University Press, 1981.
9. Burchiel KJ: Effects of electrical and mechanical stimuli on two foci of spontaneous activity which develop in primary afferent neurons after peripheral axotomy. Pain 18:249, 1984.
10. Cady L, Bischoff D, O'Connel E: Strength and fitness and subsequent back injuries in firefighters. Occup Med 21:269, 1979.
11. Carew TJ, Ghez C: Muscles and muscle receptors. In Kandel ER, Schwartz JH (eds): Principles of Neural Science. New York, Elsevier, 1985, p. 443.
12. Carpenter M: Human Neuroanatomy, 7th ed. Baltimore, Williams & Wilkins, 1976.
13. Cuello AC, Del Fiacco M, Paxinos G: The central and peripheral ends of the substance P containing sensory neurons in the rat trigeminal system. Brain Res 152:499, 1978.
14. Cyriax J: Textbook of Orthopaedic Medicine, vol. 1. London, Bailliere Tindall, 1978.
15. Dubner R, Bennet, GJ: Spinal and trigeminal mechanisms of nociception. Ann Rev Neurosci 6:381, 1983.
16. Farfan HF: Mechanical Disorders of the Lowback. Philadelphia, Lea & Febiger, 1973.
17. Feinstein B, Langton JNK, Jameson RM, Schiller F: Experiments on pain referred from deep structures. J Bone Joint Surg (Am) 36A:981, 1954.
18. Goodwin GM, McCloskey DL, Matthews PB: The contribution of muscle afferents to kinaesthesia shown by vibration induced illusions of movement and by the effects of paralysing joint afferents. Brain 95:705, 1972.
19. Goodwin GM, McCloskey DL, Matthews PB: The persistence of appreciable kinesthesia after paralysing joint afferents by preserving muscle afferents. Brain Res 37:326, 1972.
20. Gowitzke BA, Milner M: Scientific Basis of Human Movement. Baltimore, Williams & Wilkins, 1988.
21. Grieve G: Referred pain. In Grieve G (ed): Modern Manual Therapy of the Vertebral Column. Edinburgh, Churchill Livingstone, 1986, p. 233.
22. Hasue M, Kikuchi S, Sakuyama Y, Ito T: Anatomic study of the interrelation between lumbosacral nerve roots and their surrounding tissues. Spine 8:50, 1983.
23. Hirsch C, Inglemark B, Miller M: The anatomical basis for lowback pain. Acta Orthop Scand 33:1, 1963.
24. Hollinshead WH, Rosse C: Textbook of Human Anatomy. Philadelphia, Harper & Row, 1985.
25. Howe JF, Loeser JD, Calvin WH: Mechanosensitivity of dorsal root ganglia and chronically injured axons: A physiological basis for the radicular pain of nerve root compression. Pain 3:25, 1977.
26. Ikari C: A study of the mechanism of lowback pain. A neurohistological examination of the disease (abstr). J Bone Joint Surg 36A:195, 1954.
27. Kellgren JH: Observations on referred pain arising from muscle. Clin Sci 3:175, 1938.
28. Kelly JP: Reactions of neurons to injury. In Kandel E, Schwartz J (eds): Principles of Neural Science. New York, Elsevier, 1985, p. 187.
29. Lembeck F: Sir Thomas Lewis' nocifensor system, histamine and substance P containing primary afferent nerves. Trends Neurosci 6:106, 1983.
30. Lieberman AR: Sensory ganglia. In Landon DN (ed): The Peripheral Nerve, p. 182. London, Chapman & Hall, 1976.
31. Lippit AB: The facet joint and its role in spine pain. Spine 9:746, 1984.
32. Loeser JD: Pain due to nerve injury. Spine 10:232, 1985.
33. Louis R: Vertebroradicular and vertebromedullar dynamics. Anat Clin 3:1, 1981.
34. MacNab I: The mechanism of spondylogenic pain. In Hirsch C, Zotterman Y (eds): Cervical Pain. Oxford, Pergamon, 1972, p. 89.
35. Maitland G: Vertebral Manipulation, 5th ed. London, Butterworth, 1986.
36. Malinsky J: The ontogenetic development of nerve terminations in the intervertebral discs of man. Acta Anat (Basel) 38:96, 1959.
37. Martin JH: Receptor physiology and submodality coding in the somatic sensory system. In Kandel ER, Schwartz JH (eds): Principles of Neural Science. New York, Elsevier, 1985, p. 301.
38. Matthews PB: Where does Sherrington's "muscular sense" originate? Muscles, joints, corollary discharges? Annu Rev Neurosci 5:189, 1982.
39. McCall IW, Park WM, O'Brien JP: Induced pain referral from posterior lumbar elements in normal subjects. Spine 4:441, 1979.
40. McCarron RF, Wimpee MW, Hudkins PG, Laros GS: The inflammatory effect of the nucleus pulposus: A possible element in the pathogenesis of lowback pain. Spine 12:760, 1987.

41. Mixter WJ, Barr JS: Rupture of the intervertebral disc with involvement of the spinal canal. N Engl J Med 211:210, 1934.

42. Mooney V, Robertson J: The facet syndrome. Clin Orthop 115:149, 1976.

43. Morris EW, DiPaola M, Vallance R, Waddell G: Diagnosis and decision making in lumbar disc prolapse and nerve entrapment. Spine 11:436, 1986.

44. Parke WW, Watanabe R: The intrinsic vasculature of the lumbosacral nerve roots. Spine 10:508, 1985.

45. Rauschung W: Normal and pathologic anatomy of the lumbar root canals. Spine 12:1008, 1987.

46. Report of the Quebec Task Force: Scientific approach to the assessment and management of activity-related spinal disorders. Spine 12(7S):S-16, 1987.

47. Rowinski M: Afferent neurobiology of the joint. In Gould JA (ed): Orthopaedic and Sports Physical Therapy. 2nd ed. St Louis, CV Mosby, 1990, p. 49.

48. Rydevik B, Brown M, Lundborg G: Pathoanatomy and pathophysiology of nerve root compression. Spine 9:7, 1984.

49. Rydevik D, Holm S, Brown MD, Lundborg H: Nutrition of the spinal nerve roots: The role of diffusion from the cerebral spinal fluid. Trans Orthop Res Soc 9:276, 1984.

50. Schwartz JH: The cytology of neurons. In Kandel ER, Schwartz JH (eds): Principles of Neural Science, 2nd ed. New York, Elsevier, 1985, p. 27.

51. Smyth J, Wright V: Sciatica and the intervertebral disc, an experimental study. J Bone Joint Surg {Am} 40A:1401, 1959.

52. Spencer DL, Irwin GS, Miller JAA: Anatomy and significance of fixation of the lumbosacral nerve roots in sciatica. Spine 8:672, 1983.

53. Sunderland S: Avulsion of nerve roots. Handbook of Clinical Neurology, vol. 25. In Vinken PJ, Bruyn GW (eds): Injuries of the Spine and Spinal Cord, pt 1, ch. 16. New York, Elsevier, 1975, p. 1.

54. Sunderland S: Nerves and Nerve Injuries, 2nd ed. Edinburgh, Churchill Livingstone, 1978, ch. 4.

55. Sunderland S: Traumatized nerves, roots and ganglia: Musculoskeletal factors and neuropathological consequences. In Korr IM (ed): Neurobiologic Mechanisms of Manipulative Therapy. New York, Plenum Press, 1978, p. 137.

56. Vanderlinden RG: Subarticular entrapment of the dorsal root ganglion as a cause of sciatic pain. Spine 9:19, 1984.

57. Watson J: Pain and nociception—mechanisms and modulation. In Grieve G (ed): Modern Manual Therapy of the Vertebral Column. London, Churchill Livingstone, 1986, p. 206.

58. Weinstein J: Mechanisms of spinal pain: The dorsal root ganglion as a mediator of low-back pain. Spine 11:999, 1986.

59. Wyke B: Neurological aspects of lowback pain. In Jayson (ed): The Lumbar Spine and Back Pain. New York, Grune & Stratton, 1976, p. 189.

60. Yoshizawa H, O'Brien JP, Smith WT, Trumper M: The neuropathology of intervertebral discs removed for lowback pain. J Pathol 132:95, 1980.

3

STRUCTURAL AND FUNCTIONAL CONSIDERATIONS OF THE LUMBOPELVIC MUSCULATURE

MUSCLE STRUCTURE

Skeletal muscle is one of the most complex of all musculoskeletal soft tissues. It consists of muscle cells, muscle-specific extracellular matrix, and an elaborate network of nerves and vessels. Normal muscle function depends not only on the integrity of the muscle cells, but also on the nerve and vessel networks and appropriate mechanical loading.[44] In order to better understand the function of muscle, structure should be reviewed. Once structure is better understood, generalizations regarding the diverse roles of muscle can be considered. From this general framework of reference, in-

ferences regarding the specific functions of the lumbopelvic musculature can then be developed.

Muscle is constructed of various proteins of which actin and myosin represent about 84 per cent of the total.[25] The proteins form a unit that has the ability to shorten, lengthen, and vary its state of stiffness (stiffness = resistance to deformation) on demand of the central nervous system.

Actin is a double helix protein with the troponin and tropomyosin proteins located within it. Actin surrounds the larger myosin protein in a hexagonal manner (Fig. 3–1). Myosin contains cross bridges that are the linkage points

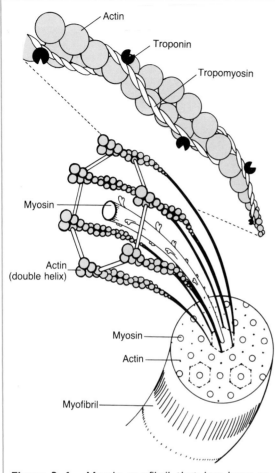

Figure 3–1. Muscle myofibril that has been reduced to its molecular form, i.e., actin (troponin, tropomysium) and myosin with cross bridges.

tween two Z lines (Fig. 3–2). Sarcomeres are placed end to end to form muscle filaments. The filaments are grouped together to form myofibrils, which in turn are further organized into groups to form muscle fibers and then organized into a specific muscle (Fig. 3–3). The magnitude of this structural complex is noted by Vander and associates,[42] who state that a "single muscle fiber 100 μm. in diameter and 1 centimeter long contains about 8,000 myofibrils, each myofibril consisting of 4500 sarcomeres. This results in a total of 16 billion thick and 64 billion thin filaments in a single fiber."

The connective tissue covering of a muscle fiber is the endomysium. Groups of muscle fibers are further organized into bundles or fasciculi that are also encased in a connective tissue covering called the perimysium. Finally, the connective tissue that covers the complete muscle is known as the epimysium (Fig. 3–4). The various connective tissues of the muscle become fused together at the terminal ends of the muscle and form a parallel arrangement of specialized connective tissue termed the tendon. Intimately related to the structural arrangement of muscle and tendon are specialized receptors known as the muscle spindle and the Golgi tendon organ. These receptors communicate the status of the muscle and tendon to the central nervous system by way of afferent nerve fibers (see Chapter 2).

MUSCLE CONTRACTION

Muscle contraction is a complex activity that involves interplay between the nervous, muscular, and skeletal systems. Because muscle contraction depends on signals from the central nervous system, its physiology is detailed below, starting at the anterior horn cell.

The cell body of a motor neuron located in the anterior horn of the spinal cord gives rise to an axon, which exits the central nervous system and travels peripherally to innervate skeletal muscle fibers. This axon, or nerve fiber, has numerous terminal branches that then innervate different muscle fibers. Through this branching network, a single nerve innervates many individual muscle fi-

between the actin and myosin proteins, and the interaction between these two proteins permits the actin to slide over the myosin.[25] This mechanism is described below.

When viewed under low magnification, the skeletal muscle appears as alternating dark and light bands owing to the configuration and overlap of the various proteins of the muscle. Attached to the sarcolemma of the cell is the Z line, which helps to physically stabilize the muscle cell. The functional unit of the muscle cell, the sarcomere, is the repeating unit be-

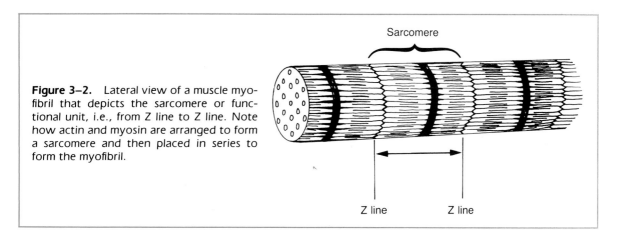

Figure 3–2. Lateral view of a muscle myofibril that depicts the sarcomere or functional unit, i.e., from Z line to Z line. Note how actin and myosin are arranged to form a sarcomere and then placed in series to form the myofibril.

bers. The motor nerve and the muscle fibers that it innervates are referred to as a motor unit. For some muscles the ratio of muscle fibers to nerve is large, whereas in others it is quite small. For example, the precise control of the eye muscles requires that one neuron control only 10 to 15 muscle fibers; in larger mus-

cles, such as the gluteus maximus, one neuron may control 2,000 to 3,000 muscle fibers. The difference in the various ratios allows for varying degrees of precision available to the muscle.

The action potential travels distally along the axon of the efferent motor neuron until it

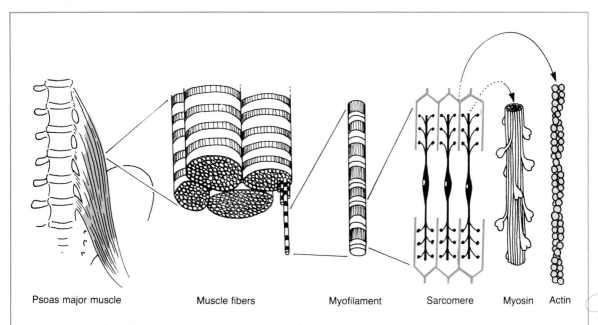

Psoas major muscle　　　　Muscle fibers　　　　Myofilament　　　　Sarcomere　　　Myosin　Actin

Figure 3–3. A progression of the structure of the muscle beginning with the actin (small filament) and myosin (large filament) molecule, progressing toward the muscle myofibril (grouped filaments), to a group of four muscle fibers (grouped myofibrils) and then to the psoas major muscle.

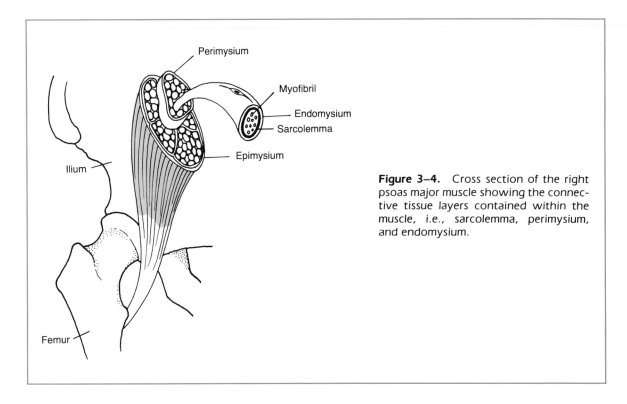

Figure 3–4. Cross section of the right psoas major muscle showing the connective tissue layers contained within the muscle, i.e., sarcolemma, perimysium, and endomysium.

reaches the presynaptic membrane at the neuromuscular junction. The neuromuscular junction is the interface between the nerve and muscle that forms the motor end-plate. Here the electrical impulse is converted to a chemical stimulus by neurotransmitters that are stored in the presynaptic membrane. Acetylcholine is the principal neurotransmitter released into the cleft of the neuromuscular junction. When acetylcholine combines with receptors in the postsynaptic membrane of the muscle fiber, the permeability of the fiber to sodium and potassium is altered. The resultant changes in the intracellular and extracellular ion concentrations cause the muscle cell membrane to be depolarized.

The frequency of this synaptic transmission can be modulated by other neurotransmitters, such as epinephrine and enkephalin.[20] The modulation also depends on other factors, such as the temporal and spatial summation of the impulses traversing the efferent motor nerve. Once depolarization occurs at the postsynaptic membrane, it is rapidly conducted across the surface of the muscle cell and into the muscle fiber by way of the transverse tubule system (T tubules). The action potential travels past sleevelike structures known as the sarcoplasmic reticulum that surround the myofibril (Fig. 3–5). Calcium is stored in the lateral sacs of the sarcoplasmic reticulum.

Excitation of the sarcoplasmic reticulum membrane triggers the release of the calcium into the contractile proteins of the muscle. The initial effect of this activity influences two of the regulatory proteins bound to actin: troponin and tropomyosin. Calcium interacts with the troponin protein that resides on the actin molecule. As the troponin is activated by the release of calcium, it changes shape and essentially pulls tropomyosin, which is situated end to end along the actin molecule, partially covering a binding site, away from the myosin binding site so that attachments between actin and myosin can develop.

At the attachment of myosin to actin a breakdown of adenosine triphosphate (ATP) to adenosine diphosphate (ADP) and inorganic

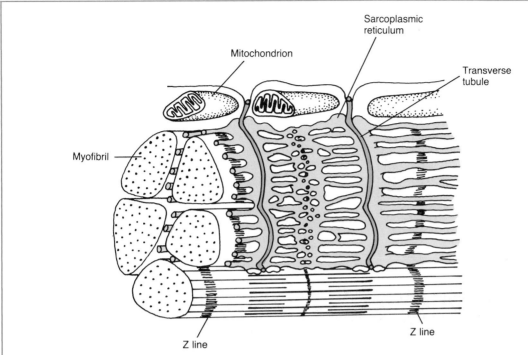

Figure 3–5. Side view of a muscle showing the sarcoplasmic reticulum and the T tubule system. These structures within the muscle complex are responsible for the conduction of the motor efferent depolarization to the muscle and the introduction of calcium into the contractile mechanism.

phosphate takes place, releasing the energy stored in ATP. This energy release results in a force that causes a movement or swiveling of the myosin cross bridge, which effectively creates a sliding of the actin over the myosin.[19] The amount of calcium released determines the number of active sites that are available for the cross bridges to develop.

As the actin slides over the myosin, the myofibril shortens. The force developed by the sliding mechanism is transmitted across the Z line to the connective tissue matrix of the muscle into the tendon and then into the bone. This connective matrix has an individually variant elasticity, a property that ultimately affects the efficiency of the contractile mechanism and the muscle's ability to meet tension requirements. This physical property of muscle is known as series elasticity (Fig. 3–6).[42]

NEUROMUSCULOSKELETAL INTEGRATION

As mentioned earlier and in Chapter 2, the muscular system is under the direct control of the central nervous system. This has important implications. The muscular system is influenced by the afferent input received by the central nervous system from the various receptors. This receptor input comes from a variety of sources, including the muscle spindles, Golgi tendon organs, and skin, joint capsule, and ligament mechanoreceptors. This afferent receptor information helps to regulate efferent motor output.

Most descriptions of muscle activity concentrate on the analysis of movement during a concentric contraction that brings the insertion of the muscle toward the origin. In addi-

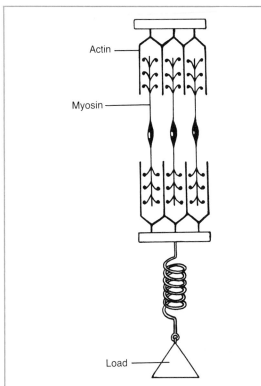

Figure 3–6. Series elastic component of the muscle. The muscle contraction (actin sliding on myosin) tenses the connective tissue matrix of the muscle (spring) (see Fig. 3–4) to impart a force to the bone, resulting in movement. The elastic qualities of the connective tissue matrix play a role in the efficiency of the muscle contraction, i.e., the more elastic the connective tissue with the muscle and tendon, the more the muscle must contract in order to impart the force to the bone.

forces through tissues that are designed to absorb and transfer them. In addition, muscles themselves can act as shock absorbers. If the neuromuscular control for these functions were not present, probably we could not perform coordinated movements, especially those associated with increased external loads, without tissue injury.

A healthy muscular system helps to assure a nondestructive load-bearing pattern through the tissues by continually adjusting to the variety of forces it is subjected to. As muscles fatigue, control or coordination of the load-bearing process is altered.[2,30] The uncontrolled loading of spinal tissues, either by single impact or prolonged overloading, increases the potential for injury. Muscle action that is controlled by afferent and efferent neuromodulation[35] results in dynamic stabilization, which plays a role in the way in which the musculoskeletal system adapts to the asymmetrical loads of movement.

The muscles of the trunk function as prime movers and stabilizers of the spine. Stabilizing or controlling the load-bearing pattern is impossible without a continuous barrage of afferent information from the environment. The afferent neural input is channeled into the central nervous system and processed to influence motor output. It is only then that contraction in correct muscle sequence becomes possible.

The central nervous system in effect "sets" the muscle for the appropriate action as a result of the afferent input. This muscle activity is typically controlled by the spinal cord, brain stem, cerebellum, and cerebral cortex. Training and reconditioning programs not only initiate anatomical and biochemical changes in muscle, but also affect the central nervous system.

✳MECHANICS OF MUSCLE

To assist in understanding the role of the musculature in the lumbopelvic unit, the mechanical nature of muscle must be considered. Muscle tension has been compared with the physical properties of springs (Fig. 3–7).[7] This is

tion to this function, muscle also contracts eccentrically and isometrically in a controlled manner that depends on both afferent feedback to the central nervous system and efferent output to the muscles. All types of muscle contraction not only affect the movement of the bone, but also generate forces to the intramuscular fascia (perimysium and endomysium), the extramuscular fascia (muscular septa and thoracolumbar fascia), the tendon, and the periosteum. Muscle activity directs

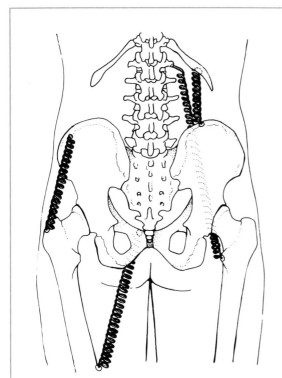

Figure 3–7. Posterior view of the lumbopelvic region showing the right quadratus lumborum muscle, right iliopsoas muscle, left gluteus medius muscle, and left femoral adductor muscles as springs replicating a mechanical model of lumbopelvic stability.

As the spring is stretched, the tension within the spring increases. Stiffness of the spring is a function of the difference in the length over the difference in the tension. In other words, as the spring is stretched, a resistance or stiffness develops by virtue of the increase in length.

Muscles behave in the same manner as they are passively or actively stretched, or as the efferent activity to the muscle is increased. The muscle has a resting tension, sometimes referred to as muscle tone, that is under direct influence of the central nervous system. This resting tension is equivalent to stiffness. The efferent output of the central nervous system increases or decreases the muscle's resting tension, depending on the summation of excitatory and inhibitory activity within the central nervous system. Excess stiffness can also lead to pathological states of motor behavior, such as rigidity and spasticity; however, these central nervous system disorders are beyond the scope of this text.

Excitatory and inhibitory balance is directly influenced by the receptor system. For example, a key function of the gamma motor system is to shorten the muscle spindle, thereby increasing the sensitivity to length changes that occur in the muscle. As another example, injury to any structure within the lumbopelvic region increases the nociceptive afferent input into the central nervous system, which may result in a new (enhanced) set point of muscle tension that can cause a resistance to movement.

Muscle tension or stiffness also increases when the muscle is stretched. For example, when a person bends forward and to the left side, the musculature on the right side of the lumbopelvic region is elongated, and an eccentric muscle contraction helps to control the movement. At the same time, the muscle must maintain a functional length in order to allow it to effectively contract concentrically and assist in returning the spine to an upright position (Fig. 3–8).

The central nervous system can alter muscle tension produced or the force output by varying the number of fibers contracting and the tension produced by that muscle fiber. The number of contracting fibers is proportional to the number of motor units activated and the

a useful analogy because it provides us with an understanding of how the various muscles, with their size, fiber direction, and contractile capabilities, might contribute to lumbopelvic stability.

Springs are mechanical devices with stored energy. From an engineering perspective, they have a certain stiffness. Stiffness can be defined as a resistance to deformation; that is, the greater the degree of stiffness of the spring, the more difficult it is to change the spring's shape. Increasing the stiffness of a structure makes it more difficult for an outside force to deform the structure. The energy from this outside force would instead be stored as potential energy.

A spring also has the ability to restore itself to its original length after it has been stretched.

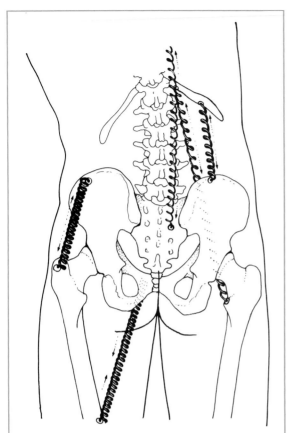

Figure 3–8. Posterior view showing the lengthening of the right posterior lumbar muscles and left pelvic muscles shown as springs as the trunk is forward bent and side bent to the left. Note the different states of muscle contraction (isometric, concentric, and eccentric) that must take place in each muscle as the trunk moves in this direction.

tion potential frequency or the frequency-tension relation. This variable relates to time delay between the contraction stimulus and the muscle contraction. As the frequency of the action potential increases, the level of muscle tension increases to the point of maximal achievable tension.

The second variable that determines muscle tension is the length-tension relation of the muscle. Every muscle has an optimal length at which it can produce the maximal amount of tension. The further the muscle length is from this optimal point, the less tension it is able to produce with contraction.

The third variable is the duration of the activity and degree of fatigue. The longer the time required for the muscle to contract, the less its ability to maintain or produce muscle tension. The exact causes of fatigue are unknown, but recent studies suggest that the excitation coupling reaction at the cross bridge may be the site of certain types of fatigue.[2]

The last variable that determines muscle tension is related to the type of muscle fiber. Different fiber types produce different amounts of muscle tension. For example, type II fibers produce greater tension but have decreased endurance capabilities. Conversely, type I aerobic fibers produce lower amounts of tension but have greater endurance capabilities.

MUSCLE TENSION RELATED TO FORCE ATTENUATION

The physical properties of the muscles that surround the spine control the manner in which forces are transferred and absorbed by the axial skeleton. The ability of the muscle to dynamically produce tension to stabilize a specific body segment so that another body part can move has significant clinical relevance, especially when developing a treatment plan for the injured patient (see Chapter 6).

The resting state of muscle stiffness (resting tension) and the ability of the central nervous system to continually alter the set-point of muscle tension in response to changing loads (active tension) are the key aspects of dynamic

number of fibers within each motor unit. Recruitment of the motor neurons depends on the load that must be overcome. The size principle[42] states that the smaller motor units initially contract and are followed by the contraction of the larger motor units to increase total muscle tension. As the load increases, greater muscle tension is required to move the load and a greater number of fibers must contract.

Tension produced by the muscle contraction depends on four variables.[42] The first is the ac-

stabilization. The muscle's attachments and the effect that resting tension and active tension have on intervening tissues because of these attachments are important to consider. Because of this tension, the muscle can act as a true shock absorber in the attenuation of ground and trunk forces. The functional implication is that the muscle with an enhanced setpoint is more reactive to a given stimulus, and the increased stiffness allows it to be more effective as a shock absorber.

Injury can occur when the contractile and noncontractile tissues are unable to control the forces of gravity and movement and the viscoelastic capacity of the tissues is exceeded. Forces applied with sufficiently great magnitude and speed, or a lesser force imparted over an excessive period of time, can render the connective tissue matrix vulnerable to disruption and minimize the ability of the tissue to stabilize the bony segments. Once deformation or structural alteration of the connective tissue takes place, excessive or abnormal movements can occur between spinal segments if the muscles are unable to stabilize the area. Altered mechanics can cause further deformation of the tissues, and if tissue damage results, the nociceptor system is activated.

It is important for the clinician dealing with mechanical low back pain to understand the relations between contractile and noncontractile tissues in the lumbopelvic region. The lumbopelvic anatomy should be readily visualized in order to assess the tensile, compressive, torsional, and shear forces directed into and through the tissues during movement.

Without a three-dimensional appreciation of the functional anatomy of this region, effective evaluation and treatment of the low back are difficult. Once the clinician gains an understanding of the functional anatomy of the trunk, logical and effective treatment programs can be implemented.

FUNCTIONAL ANATOMY OF THE LUMBOPELVIC REGION

One of the best examples of the intricacies of neuromuscular regulation mechanisms is the lumbopelvic complex, which requires an integration of the musculature of the lumbar spine, pelvis, and hips. This section of the chapter examines the muscles of the lumbopelvic region and explores their contribution to the stability and control required to permit smooth motion and prevent sprain and strain. The muscles and related connective tissues of the lumbar spine are described much in the same way that they would be encountered in a dissection of the lumbar spine. After this, the musculature of both the abdominal wall and the hip is reviewed, since it has a profound influence on lumbopelvic mechanics. The articulations of the lumbopelvic region, intervertebral disc, sacroiliac joint, pubic symphysis, and hip joint are discussed in Chapter 4.

Thoracolumbar Fascia

The first structure encountered when the skin and subcutaneous fat are removed from the posterior aspect of the lumbar spine is the thoracolumbar fascia (Fig. 3–9). The thoracolumbar fascia forms a network of noncontractile tissue that plays an essential role in the function of the lumbar spine.

In the lumbar region the fascia can be divided into posterior, middle, and anterior layers. The posterior layer is a thick, fibrous covering that can be subdivided into two lamellae.[4] This layer is attached to the spinous processes and the supraspinous ligament and continues laterally over the erector spinae muscle to converge into the lateral raphe (Fig. 3–10). At this juncture the fascia turns anterior and medial to surround the erector spinae and multifidus muscles. As it continues medially, it attaches to the transverse processes and the intertransverse ligaments of the lumbar vertebrae. This medial continuation of the fascial layer attaching to the transverse processes forms the middle layer of thoracolumbar fascia.

From the lateral raphe the fascia also extends further anteriorly to surround the quadratus lumborum muscle, and laterally to attach to the transverse abdominis and internal oblique muscles. Inferiorly, the thoracolumbar fascia also has attachments to the sacrum and

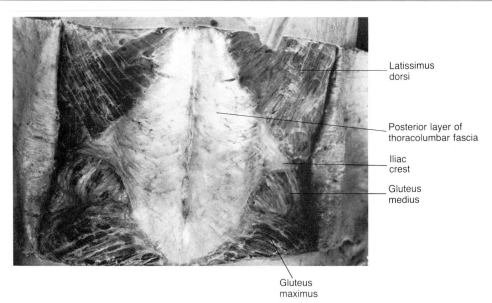

Latissimus dorsi

Posterior layer of thoracolumbar fascia

Iliac crest

Gluteus medius

Gluteus maximus

Figure 3–9. Posterior view of a cadaveric specimen with the skin and subcutaneus fat removed, showing the latissimus dorsi muscle and the gluteus maximus muscle as they attach to the posterior layer of the thoracolumbar fascia.

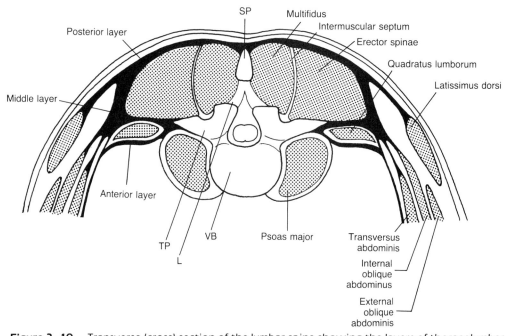

SP

Multifidus

Intermuscular septum

Posterior layer

Erector spinae

Quadratus lumborum

Latissimus dorsi

Middle layer

Anterior layer

TP

VB

L

Psoas major

Transversus abdominis

Internal oblique abdominus

External oblique abdominus

Figure 3–10. Transverse (cross) section of the lumbar spine showing the layers of thoracolumbar fascia (posterior, middle, and anterior) and the muscles attached to it and contained within it. Also labeled are the spinous process (SP), transverse process (TP), vertebral body (VB), and lamina (L). The juncture of the posterior and middle layers is the lateral raphe.

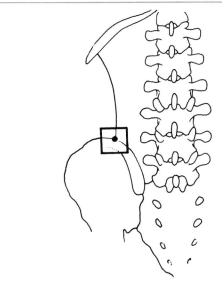

Figure 3–11. Inferiormost aspect of the attachment of the lateral raphe. A significant anchor point to the pelvis that includes thoracolumbar fascia, tendons of the superficial and deep iliocostalis lumborum muscle, and the lateral aspect of the iliolumbar ligament.

to the guy wires of a tent that are used to tighten and secure the structure (Fig. 3–13). As the guy wires of the tent are pulled tight and secured, the tent assumes its shape and becomes stable enough to perform its function of providing a rigid structure for shelter. Similarly, as the body moves, muscular forces internal and external to the thoracolumbar fascia potentially afford the same type of stabilizing function.

Tension can thus be imparted to the fascia actively or passively.[39] Contraction of the latissimus dorsi, internal oblique, or transversus abdominis can exert a tensile force to the thoracolumbar fascia. By virtue of the direct attachments of these muscles, an active tensile force results. Contraction of the posterior thigh or abdominal muscles that causes posterior rotation of the pelvis also tightens the thoracolumbar fascia. Flexion of the lumbar spine on the pelvis as in forward bending similarly results in tightening of the fascia. In these latter two instances, tension is placed on the fascia indirectly because of the lumbar flexion motion, which results in passive engagement of the fascia.

ilium, where it blends with the fascia of the gluteus maximus.

The attachment of the lateral raphe to the iliac crest is in the same location as the inferior attachment of the erector spinae aponeurosis and the deep erector spinae muscles (Fig. 3–11). Potential stresses to this region should be recognized, especially when evaluating the mechanics of forward bending.

The thoracolumbar fascia, although noncontractile tissue, can be engaged dynamically because of the contractile tissues attached to it and contained within it (Fig. 3–12A and B).[8,34] The dynamics of this tissue network can be compared to the stabilization of a tent. The central pole of the tent compares to the erector spinae, multifidus, and quadratus lumborum muscles. These muscles are contained within the fascia or "tent," and the contraction that results in broadening of the muscle exerts a pushing force on the fascia.[10] The latissimus dorsi, gluteus maximus, transversus abdominis, and internal oblique muscles are similar

Latissimus Dorsi Muscle

At first inspection it would not appear that the latissimus dorsi muscle, usually described as an extensor, adductor, and medial rotator of the humerus, has a significant effect on lumbopelvic mechanics. However, its attachments warrant its consideration as a muscle that has the potential to influence these mechanics.

Hollinshead and Rosse[17] describe the attachment of the muscle to the lower six thoracic spinous processes and all of the spinous processes of the lumbar vertebrae and sacrum through the fascial network of the thoracolumbar fascia. The relation to the thoracolumbar fascia is further described below. The inferior attachment of the latissimus dorsi muscle continues laterally along the iliac crest toward the point of attachment of the lateral raphe of the thoracolumbar fascia and the erector spinae aponeurosis. From these points of attachment the muscle converges upward and laterally to

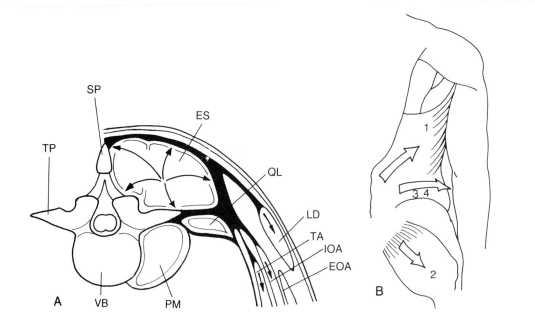

Figure 3–12. *A*, Transverse section of the lumbar spine depicting the forces imparted to the thoracolumbar fascia by contraction of muscles that are attached to it and are contained within it. Spinous process (SP), transverse process (TP), vertebral body (VB), erector spinae muscle (ES), latissimus dorsi muscle (LD), quadratus lumborum muscle (QL), internal oblique muscle (IOA), transversus abdominis muscle (TA). *B*, Posterior view of the musculature that attaches to the thoracolumbar fascia. Note the forces that are generated to the fascia from the latissimus dorsi muscle (1) from above, the gluteus maximus muscle (2) from below, and the internal oblique abdominis muscle (3) and transversus abdominis muscle (4) from the front.

attach to the lesser tubercle of the humerus and the floor of the intertubercular groove.

On the deep surface of the latissimus dorsi muscle there is a distinct layer of fascia. When

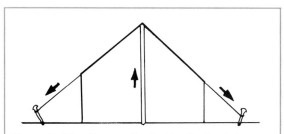

Figure 3–13. Forces directed to the fascia by various muscles are similar to those encountered when erecting a tent. The direction and forces exerted by the guy wires directly affect the stability of the tent.

this deep fascia is followed to the muscle's lateral border, it is found to fuse with the fascial layer on the superficial surface of the muscle. Medially, the fascia covering the latissimus dorsi muscle fuses with the aponeurotic origin of the muscle where a dense, thick contribution is made to the thoracolumbar fascia.

Because the lumbopelvic attachment of the latissimus dorsi muscle is by way of the thoracolumbar fascia, a relation to spine mechanics can be contemplated. McGill and Norman[26] note that when all of the posterior trunk tissues are considered, the latissimus dorsi muscle has the largest moment arm length. This implies that the latissimus dorsi muscle potentially influences lumbopelvic mechanics with less effort than do other tissues because of this mechanical advantage.

Before considering the force vector that this

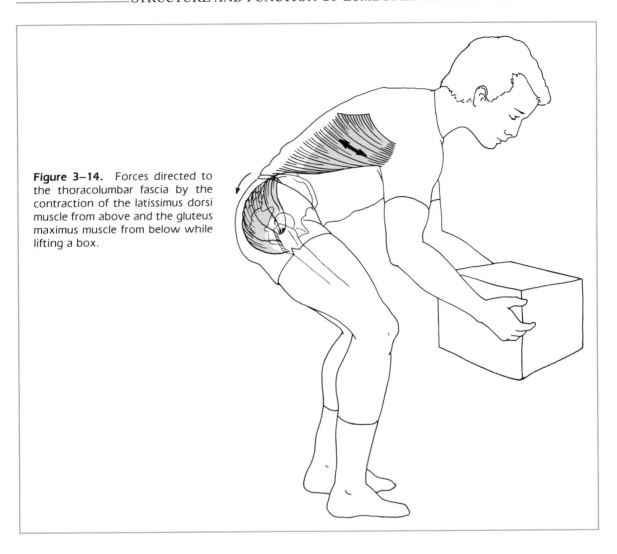

Figure 3–14. Forces directed to the thoracolumbar fascia by the contraction of the latissimus dorsi muscle from above and the gluteus maximus muscle from below while lifting a box.

muscle exerts on the thoracolumbar fascia, it should be noted that the position of the humerus influences the thoracolumbar fascia. If the humerus is in an abducted and flexed position, as is typical for a person reaching for an object to lift or pull toward the body, the muscle is stretched. If there is concurrent posterior rotation of the pelvis, the tensile force to the fascia is further enhanced. If the latissimus dorsi muscle is now called on to contract, then an active tensile force is also imparted to the fascia (Fig. 3–14).

The latissimus dorsi muscle is not typically viewed as a lifting muscle. A kinematic analysis of the lifting task suggests that the latissimus dorsi muscle appears capable of helping to overcome the inertia of the object as one attempts to move it closer to the body. When functional lift tasks are scrutinized, it is apparent that the latissimus dorsi muscle assists in moving the load closer to the subject's center of gravity. As the lift continues, the angle between the humerus and the body changes. Note that it is possible to lift or move the weight toward the body without significant latissimus dorsi contribution. With only a strong spinal extensor contraction and the subject's hands firmly grasping the object, the weight can be accelerated by spinal extensor muscle action, which can also overcome the inertia of the stationary object. The upper limbs then move passively toward the subject's trunk while the weight is held. This activity may strain the spinal extensor muscles. Although not substantiated by scientific method, it remains logical to conclude that the latissimus dorsi muscle can contribute to equalizing forces on lumbopelvic tissues.

This stabilization presumably is enhanced by muscle contraction of a new set-point of muscle tension, which in effect exerts a pull on the fascia. A bilateral pull on the fascia by both latissimus dorsi muscles has the effect of pulling on both sides of the spinous and transverse process attachments of the thoracolumbar fascia, which assists in checking rotation and flex-

ion of the lumbar spine. A contraction of the ipsilateral latissimus dorsi muscle requires a counterforce by the musculature on the contralateral side to minimize aberrant motion in the lumbar spine. The oblique and transverse abdominal muscles, for example, by virtue of their attachments and fiber direction, appear capable of providing this counterforce.[40]

Erector Spinae Muscles: The Superficial and Deep Iliocostalis Lumborum and Longissimus Thoracis Muscles

The term erector spinae is used in reference to the paraspinal muscles innervated by branches of the dorsal rami (see Chapter 2). Al-

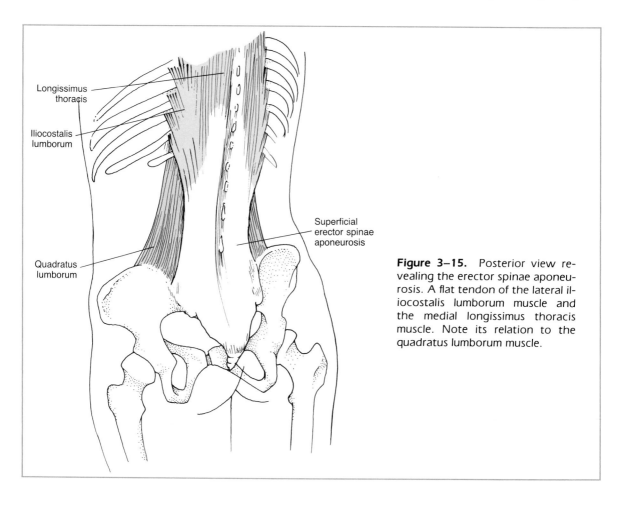

Longissimus thoracis

Iliocostalis lumborum

Quadratus lumborum

Superficial erector spinae aponeurosis

Figure 3–15. Posterior view revealing the erector spinae aponeurosis. A flat tendon of the lateral iliocostalis lumborum muscle and the medial longissimus thoracis muscle. Note its relation to the quadratus lumborum muscle.

though the erector spinae muscles traverse the complete length of the spine, this section is limited to discussing the superficial and deep iliocostalis and longissimus divisions in the lumbopelvic region.

The superficial aspects of the iliocostalis lumborum and longissimus thoracis muscles are attached to the undersurface of a broad, flat tendon and the iliac crest. The tendinous sheet of attachment is referred to as the *erector spinae aponeurosis*. This tendinous insertion continues medially along the ilium and extends to the spinous processes in the lumbar and sacral regions. The superficial erector spinae muscles arise from the anterior aspect of this aponeurosis and ascend to attach to the ribs (Fig. 3–15).

These superficial muscles have an excellent lever arm over the lumbar spine by virtue of their attachments, and function eccentrically to control the descent of the spine in forward bending, concentrically to extend the spine, and isometrically to control the position of the lower thorax with respect to the pelvis.[9,12,27,31,36,37] The erector spinae muscles have been shown to enter into a period of electromyographic silence toward the end of forward bending.[12,23,33,43] It has been proposed that at this point the stabilization of the spine has been relinquished or passed on to the noncontractile structures of the back, and that the muscle has been stretched to a length that minimizes its ability to contract.[11]

The concept of an electrically silent muscle should be interpreted with caution. It may be incorrect to assume that the electrically silent muscle is inactive. A muscle at rest still maintains a resting tension or tone. Thus even in this lengthened state, the musculature contributes to limiting further forward bending.

Bogduk[3] has described a significant deeper division of the erector spinae muscles that is distinct from the previously described superficial component. This deep, lumbar division originates from the ilium just anterior to the superficial insertion of the erector spinae aponeurosis and extends superiorly, anteriorly, and medially toward the lumbar transverse processes. The lumbar portion consists of a lateral iliocostalis attaching to the lateral aspect of the lumbar transverse processes and a me-

dial longissimus attaching to the accessory processes. An intermuscular septum separates the two divisions.[6]

The attachments of the deep portion of the erector spinae represent an important functional consideration. Figure 3–16 shows these deep attachments, which emphasizes how the lumbar vertebrae are anchored to the ilium through this muscle complex. The orientation of the deep erector spinae muscles allows for the generation of muscle force in various directions. As this muscle is followed from its caudal iliac crest attachment, the deep portion has an anterior inclination as it reaches the lower lumbar transverse and accessory processes.

In addition to extension of the lumbar spinal segments, it is reasonable to conclude that contraction of the lumbar portion of the erector spinae has additional effects on the lumbar spine. The first may be to help check or reduce

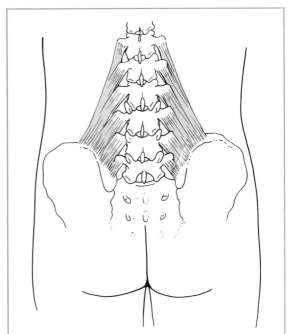

Figure 3–16. Attachments of the deep erector spinae muscles. These deep muscles function to anchor the lumbar vertebrae to the ilium. Contraction of these muscles probably stabilize rather than prime move.

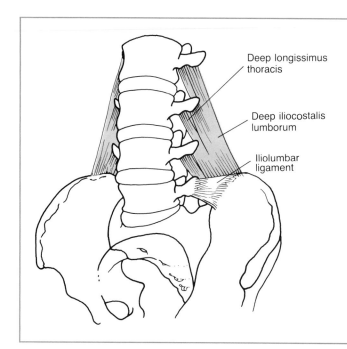

Deep longissimus thoracis

Deep iliocostalis lumborum

Iliolumbar ligament

Figure 3–17. *Anterior oblique view showing the direction of the deep erector spinae muscle. These muscles assist in reducing the anterior shear of the lumbar vertebrae and manage the lumbar lordosis, assuring proper weight-bearing. Note their relation to the iliolumbar ligament.*

anterior shear of L4 on L5 and L5 on S1 by way of its posteriorly directed force. Furthermore, the vector of the muscle action is along a line that tends to decrease the lumbar curve by a posteriorly directed force on the lumbar vertebrae (Fig. 3–17). The posterior shear force exerted by the deep portion of the erector spinae muscles acts in a direction to reduce the lumbar lordosis.

An anteroposterior (sagittal plane) guy wire or check system is thus available when considering the contraction vector of the ipsilateral psoas major muscle. Contraction of the psoas major muscle can cause an anterior shear force on the lumbar vertebrae. The deep erector spinae perhaps works with the contralateral psoas major muscle to create a sagittal plane check-and-balance system for lumbar stability (Fig. 3–18A and B).

Another function of the deep erector spinae muscles, by way of their vertical vector, may be to increase the compressive forces between vertebral segments. Compression forces, which are discussed below, are important in locking the vertebral assembly to assist with intersegmental stabilization. The direction of the vector of these muscles also helps to check rotary forces of the lumbar spine. For example, the deep portion of the erector spinae on the right presumably functions isometrically and eccentrically to control left vertebral rotation.

The erector spinae muscle thus consists of two parts. They are a superficial or costal portion and a deep or vertebral portion. Because of their attachments and orientation, these two divisions of the erector spinae have different functions as they control and move the lumbar spine.

Multifidus Muscles

The multifidus muscles are referred to in textbooks of anatomy as transversospinalis muscles. This name is chosen because muscles of this group run in a lateral to medial direction from the transverse processes to the spinous processes of the vertebrae. Unfortunately this description is inadequate for the multifidus muscles in the lumbopelvic region, especially at the L4–L5, L5–S1, and sacral regions.

In the lumbopelvic region the multifidus

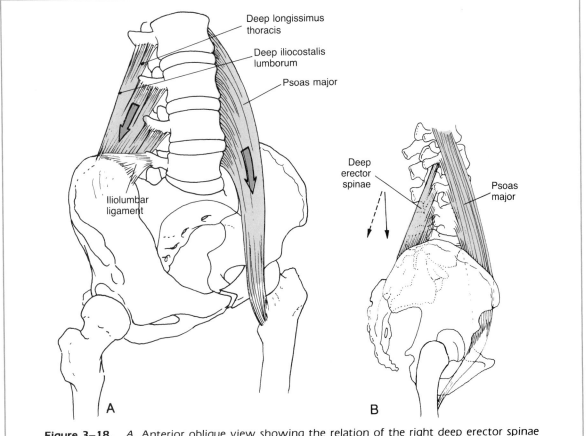

Figure 3–18. *A,* Anterior oblique view showing the relation of the right deep erector spinae muscle and the left psoas major muscle as they function together contralaterally to stabilize the lumbar spine by way of the anteroposterior guy wire check system. The arrows depict the direction of the muscular forces imparted to the lumbar spine. *B,* Sagittal view showing the stabilizing relation of the deep erector spinae muscle and psoas major muscle.

arises from the dorsal surface of the sacrum, the aponeurosis of the erector spinae muscle, the medial surface of the posterior superior iliac spine, and the posterior sacroiliac ligaments. The muscle also originates from the mammillary processes in the lumbar spine.[5,32]

From these caudal attachments the muscle runs superiorly and medially to attach to the spinous processes (Fig. 3–19). Owing to the posterior concavity of the lumbar spine and the convexity of the sacral kyphosis, the muscle also has a slight anterior inclination as it courses to attach to the lumbar spinous processes at the apex of the lordosis.

The multifidus musculature is thick and prominent in the lumbopelvic region. It fills the extensive channel bordered by the lumbar transverse and spinous processes. Owing to the size of the lumbar vertebrae, it should be apparent that this is a large muscle mass. This is not the case as the multifidus muscle is followed up the spine. The gross anatomy of the multifidus is different in the lumbopelvic region compared with that in the cervical and thoracic spine. It becomes much more compact as it is closely attached to the sides of the progressively smaller spinous processes, and the above-mentioned channel between the trans-

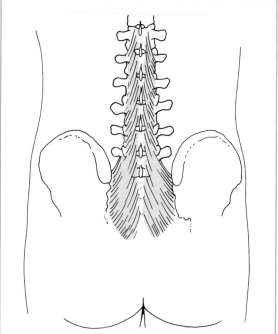

Figure 3–19. Multifidus muscle running superior and medial to attach to the spinous processes of the lumbar and sacral vertebrae.

verse processes and the spinous processes becomes progressively narrower.

The extensive attachment of the multifidus muscle to the dorsal surface of the sacrum makes it the major tissue mass filling the deep sulcus formed by the overlapping ilium and the sacrum. This sulcus is directly medial to the posterior superior iliac spine. From a palpation standpoint, tenderness in the area medial to the posterior superior iliac spine and on either side of the spinous processes may be due to irritation of this muscle tissue directly or its covering of aponeurosis and fascia (Fig. 3–20A through F). Furthermore, injury to any other innervated tissue in the lumbopelvic region may lead to excessive muscle activity or muscle guarding, which is initiated to protect the injury site from further movement. The extensive direct attachment of the multifidus muscle to the lumbar spine makes it a prime candidate for muscle guarding because of lumbar spine injury.

The attachment of the multifidus muscles to the spinous processes results in an effective lever arm for lumbar extension (Fig. 3–21). Because the axis of rotation for flexion and exten-

Figure 3–20. *See legend on opposite page.*

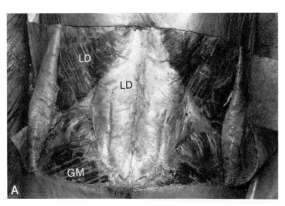

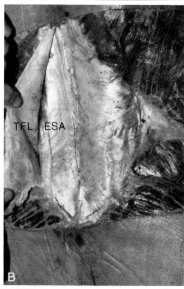

TLF = Thoracolumbar fascia
LD = Latissimus dorsi muscle
GM = Gluteus maximus muscle

ESA = Erector spinae aponeurosis
TLF = Thoracolumbar fascia
(reflected on left)

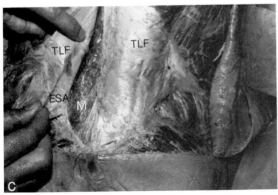

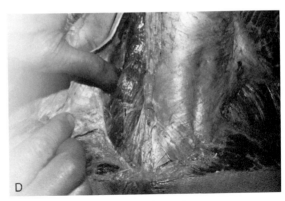

TLF = Thoracolumbar fascia (reflected on left)
ESA = Erector spinae aponeurosis (reflected on left
M = Multifidus muscle

I = Intermuscular septum

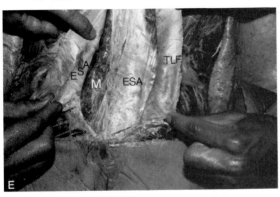

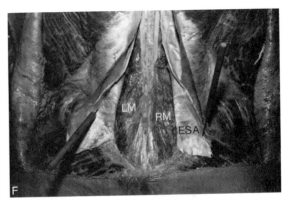

M = Multifidus
ESA = Erector spinae aponeurosis
TLF = Thoracolumbar fascia (reflected)

RM = Right multifidus muscle
LM = Left multifidus muscle
ESA = Erector spinae aponeurosis (reflected)

Figure 3–20. *A,* Thoracolumbar fascia. Posterior view of a cadaveric specimen with the skin and subcutaneous fat removed showing the superficial or posterior layer of the thoracolumbar fascia. Note the attachments of the latissimus dorsi muscle from above and the gluteus maximus muscle from below. *B,* Erector spinae aponeurosis. Posterior view (close up) revealing the posterior layer of the thoracolumbar fascia removed on the left, exposing the left erector spinae aponeurosis. Note the tendon of the medial (longissimus thoracis muscle) and lateral (iliocostalis lumborum muscle) of the superficial erector spinae muscle group. *C,* Left multifidus muscle. Same view as in *B* with the left erector spinae aponeurosis dissected and reflected lateral to reveal the left multifidus muscle. *D,* Intermuscular septum. Same view as in *B* and *C* showing the intermuscular septum (at thumb) that surrounds the left multifidus muscle. Just lateral to the septum is the deep erector spinae muscle (see Fig. 3–9). *E,* Right erector spinae aponeurosis. Posterior layer of the thoracolumbar fascia on the right is reflected away to show the right erector spinae aponeurosis. *F,* Bilateral multifidus muscles. Reflected bilaterally the posterior layer of the thoracolumbar fascia and erector spinae aponeurosis to reveal both multifidus muscles. Note the strong ligamentous extensions from the 5th lumbar spinous process to the sacrum.

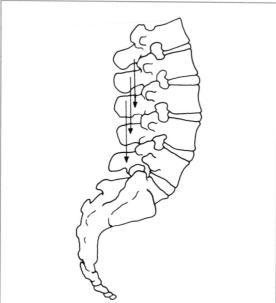

Figure 3–21. Sagittal view revealing the vector or line of pull of the multifidus muscle that makes it a strong spinal extensor. (Adapted from Bogduk N, Twomey LT: Clinical Anatomy of the Lumbar Spine. Churchill Livingstone, New York, 1987.)

sion is in the posterior region of the disc, the distance from the spinous processes to this axis is actually longer than the lever arm of the deep portions of the erector spinae, which attaches to the region of the transverse processes. It is therefore more effective in causing extension of the lumbovertebral segments.[5] From a functional standpoint, especially while in the standing position, the action of the muscle is probably antiflexion and antishear. That is, contraction by the multifidus muscles helps to control these two forces (flexion and shear) during forward bending. Contraction of the multifidus muscle places a posteriorly and inferiorly directed force on L5 and L4 that counters the anterior shear force that occurs as a result of the lumbar lordosis. This anterior shear force is also increased with forward bending postures encountered during lifting. Note that the force of the multifidus muscle is opposite that of the psoas major muscle, and they may

potentially function together to "square" the vertebral unit in the sagittal plane.

The multifidus muscle also has an oblique orientation in the frontal plane. Most anatomy textbooks state that contraction of the muscle causes rotation to the opposite side. Although this might occur, its lever arm for this activity is not optimal, and the muscle appears mechanically inefficient. It probably remains active during all antigravity activity.[9,27,41] As with the deep erector spinae muscles, contraction of the multifidus muscles exerts a compressive force between each lumbar vertebrae and between L5 and the sacrum. Stability of the lumbar spine increases when compressive forces are placed on it. When loaded in compression, the lumbopelvic unit is much more resistant to torsional forces that have the potential to damage the outer annular rings and the lumbar zygapophysial joint.[10] Therefore, the multifidus muscle may contribute to spinal stability by "squeezing" the vertebrae together and locking or engaging the vertebral assembly.

Sirca and Kostevc[38] have found more type I fibers in the multifidus muscles of the lumbar spine, which suggests that this muscle has a greater tonic or stabilizing function rather than dynamic prime mover actions. Thus, when muscle fiber type and vector analysis are considered, the multifidus muscle appears capable of assisting with stabilization of the lumbar spine. Much research needs to be done in the area of functional training of this muscle. Just as the hamstring and quadriceps muscles are trained for the unstable knee, perhaps functional training may offer treatment for segmental instability.

Intersegmental Muscles

There is a series of small muscles of the lumbopelvic region that connect one intervertebral segment with another. These muscles are typically named for the portions of the bone to which they attach. Many of their functions can only be presumed from observation of their anatomical position. They are the interspinales, which are located on either side of the interspinous ligament, and the intertransversarii

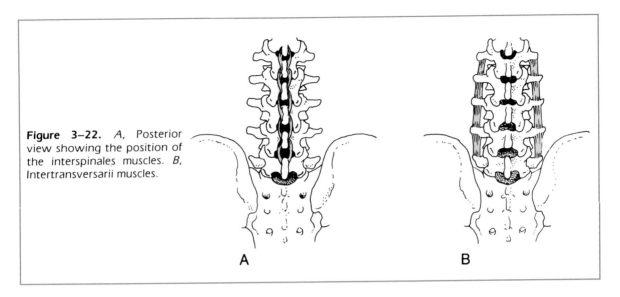

Figure 3–22. *A,* Posterior view showing the position of the interspinales muscles. *B,* Intertransversarii muscles.

A   B

muscles, which attach to adjacent mammillary and transverse processes (Fig. 3–22*A* and *B*).

The interspinales muscles are considered to be extensors of the lumbar segments, while the intertransversarii probably participate in extension and lateral flexion. The cross-sectional area of these muscles is small, and therefore the magnitude of their contribution is questionable. However, because of their attachment to each vertebra, they may be responsible for providing proprioceptive input to the central nervous system, as they are continually placed under a variety of tensile or compressive forces with activity.

Quadratus Lumborum Muscle

The quadratus lumborum muscle is usually studied with the posterior abdominal wall. When studied in this manner, its influence on lumbopelvic mechanics is seldom appreciated. However, its attachment to the lumbar spine and pelvis warrants its study as a muscle of the lumbopelvic region.

The quadratus lumborum muscle consists of fibers that are oriented in three directions.[21] The muscle can be divided into a component that extends from the iliac crest to the lumbar transverse processes (iliotransverse), another part that extends from the lumbar transverse processes to the lower ribs (costotransverse), and a final part that originates from the iliac crest and proceeds to the lower ribs (iliocostal) (Fig. 3–23). The costotransverse portion is very small and often not discernible; therefore, it is not considered in this discussion.

The quadratus lumborum occupies the region over the iliac crest just adjacent to the lateral border of the erector spinae muscles. Because the quadratus lumborum has a major attachment to the iliac crest, and the complete border of the iliac crest can often be directly palpated, it is reasonable to consider this muscle's potential involvement in painful syndromes that involve the iliac crest.

From this region the iliocostal portion of the quadratus lumborum muscle ascends superiorly and medially under cover of this thick component of the erector spinae muscle to attach to the lower ribs. The iliotransverse portion travels superiorly and medially to attach to the lateral aspect of the transverse process of the lumbar vertebrae. The latter portion is not under cover of any thick musculature, but is deep to the thoracolumbar fascia and the muscular attachments to this fascia—the internal oblique, transversus abdominis, and latissimus dorsi muscles. This anatomical relation should be considered when palpating areas of tender-

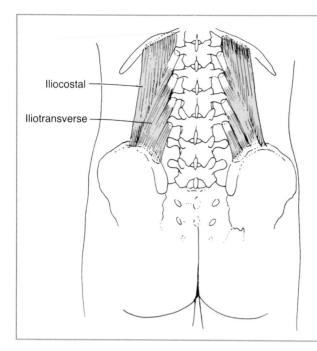

Iliocostal

Iliotransverse

Figure 3–23. Posterior view showing the quadratus lumborum muscle. This muscle has three portions, iliocostal, iliotransverse, and costotransverse. This figure does not show the costotransverse portion because it is often insignificant in its size and function and, if present, lies on the anterior aspect of the muscle. These muscles produce lateral guy wire forces to the lumbar spine.

ness, especially in relation to the muscle's attachment on the iliac crest (i.e., lateral to the iliocostalis lumborum muscle) (see Fig. 3–10).

Although one action of the muscle is to "hike" the hip, we seldom use the muscle in this manner unless we are attempting to compensate for a relatively longer limb during gait. The muscle has more important functions relative to moving and stabilizing the pelvis and lumbar spine.

For example, during a side-bending motion of the trunk from the standing position, the quadratus lumborum muscle on the convex side of the curve undergoes an eccentric contraction in order to help control the rate of descent. The return to an upright position requires a concentric contraction by the same muscle. In the upright standing posture a lateral trunk sway probably requires synchronized movements, using both eccentric and concentric contractions between the right and left quadratus lumborum muscles as well as other lumbopelvic muscles to assure postural stability. The quadratus lumborum muscle appears capable of contracting in synchrony with the opposite gluteus medius muscle and femoral adductor muscles to maintain frontal plane

stability of the pelvis and lumbopelvic joints (Fig. 3–24).

Another example of mechanical stresses imparted to this muscle occurs as the upper extremities are elevated from the side that moves the lower ribs away from the iliac crest, and the trunk is flexed. The position increases the tensile stress on the quadratus lumborum muscle from both the flexed trunk and the upper extremities. The two motions are often combined in daily activities, resulting in a near maximal elongation of the quadratus lumborum muscle. If a person is forward bending and side bending to the left in order to pull an object toward him, the right quadratus lumborum muscle is placed in a position of stretch by virtue of the elevation of the rib cage in forward bending and left lateral flexion. It is reasonable to postulate that this stretch, if excessive, or the initial concentric burst of activity as the person returns to the upright position can potentially strain the muscle.

The quadratus lumborum muscle also has actions in the horizontal plane. The attachments to the lumbar transverse processes give the muscle a reasonable lever arm in attempting to control torsion of the lumbar spine. We

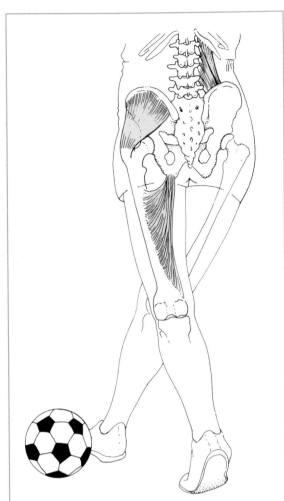

Figure 3–24. *Right quadratus lumborum muscle, left gluteus medius muscle, and left femoral adductor muscles working together to stabilize the frontal plane of the pelvis while kicking a soccer ball with the right foot. These muscular forces are necessary to assure nondestructive weight-bearing of the lumbopelvic bone and joint structures.*

plasia of the inferiormost aspect of the quadratus lumborum muscle. This is an excellent example of how the body tissues make specific adaptations to imposed demands, that is, the development of dense, fibrous tissue from a muscle in response to the forces required to stabilize the lumbosacral region.

The iliolumbar ligament has many segments that are designed to stabilize the anterior aspect of the sacroiliac joint and the L5–S1 segment.[5] A significant portion of the ligament attaches to the fifth lumbar transverse process and courses toward the ilium. This fiber direction is similar to that followed by the quadratus lumborum muscle and the deep portion of the erector spinae muscle.

The quadratus lumborum, working with such structures as the iliolumbar ligament and deep portion of the erector spinae muscles, helps to maintain stability of the lumbar spine in the frontal plane. The iliolumbar ligament "squares" or anchors the L5 vertebra down onto the S1 vertebral body.[24] This compressive force of the L5 vertebra is counteracted by the hydrophilic pressure of the L5–S1 intervertebral disk (Fig. 3–25).

Lumbar Musculature: Summary

The thoracolumbar fascia and attached latissimus dorsi muscle are superficially located over the posterior trunk. The prominent bilateral muscular ridges on the back correspond to the erector spinae and multifidus muscle groups. Just lateral to these ridges, above the level of the iliac crest, lies the quadratus lumborum muscle, which is covered by skin and the posterior layer of thoracolumbar fascia. Lateral to this point is the posterior extent of the external oblique, internal oblique, and transversus abdominis muscles. Medially the quadratus lumborum is under cover of the deep erector spinae and multifidus muscles. At the lumbosacral segment the quadratus lumborum muscle is replaced by the iliolumbar ligament. The relations of these structures must be recognized when functionally assessing the lumbopelvic region.

can again view the quadratus lumborum muscle as participating with the deep erector spinae muscle in preparing the lumbar spine for force transference.

Luk and colleagues[24] suggest that the iliolumbar ligament has developed owing to meta-

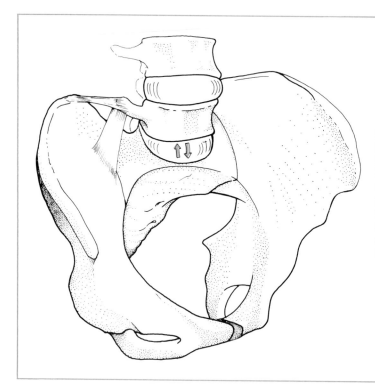

Figure 3–25. Anterior lateral view of the right iliolumbar ligament complex. Bilaterally, this ligamentous complex functions to stabilize the fifth lumbar segment against anterior shear. The iliolumbar ligament also functions with the distractive force of the L5–S1 intervertebral disc to assure L5–S1 segmental stability. The ligament, in essence, pulls the vertebral (L5) body down on the intervertebral disc.

ILIOPSOAS MUSCLES: PSOAS MAJOR AND ILIACUS MUSCLES

The psoas major muscle is attached to the anterolateral surfaces of the vertebral bodies and their respective transverse processes, and the lumbar intervertebral discs. The muscle then passes inferiorly and laterally to merge with the tendon of the iliacus muscle. The iliacus is attached superiorly to the iliac fossa and the inner lip of the iliac crest. The combined tendons then track over the superior lateral aspect of the pubic ramus and attach to the lesser trochanter of the femur (Fig. 3–26). Both the iliacus and the psoas major muscles are normally considered together, thus the term iliopsoas. This discussion reviews the muscles as a synergistic group, and then each muscle is considered individually.

The iliopsoas muscle is a flexor of the femur on the pelvis when the foot is off the ground. This action can occur when the lumbar attachment of the psoas major muscle and the pelvic attachment of the iliacus are fixed or stabilized. By keeping the lumbar spine and pelvis in a stable, nonmovable position, the femur then becomes the movable segment and flexion of the hip occurs.

The iliopsoas muscle is also a lateral rotator of the femur when the foot is free of the ground. This action can be appreciated by recognizing that in the frontal plane, the lesser trochanter is positioned posteriorly on the medial surface of the femur. Contraction of this muscle directs a force to the lesser trochanter, pulling it forward, which results in lateral rotation of the femur.

Although these actions are important, the action of the muscles when the foot is fixed on the ground should also be noted. Under these closed kinetic chain conditions the insertion at the lesser trochanter becomes the fixed end, and force occurs at the pelvis in the case of the iliacus muscle, and at the lumbar spine in the case of the psoas major muscle.

For example, when the foot is fixed on the

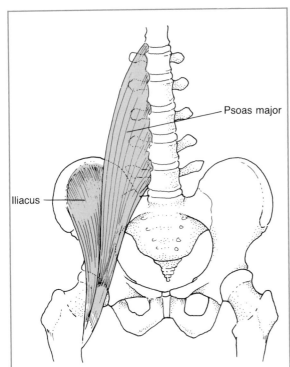

Figure 3–26. Anterior view showing the iliopsoas muscle complex containing the psoas major muscle and iliacus muscle. Note their relation to the superior ramus of the pubis and the anterior aspect of the hip joint.

The psoas major muscle has different actions than the iliacus by virtue of its lumbar attachments. Nachemson[29] has noted that this muscle is electromyographically active in many different postures and movements. Muscle activity at the vertebral attachment of this muscle may add a compressive effect on the lumbar body–intervertebral disc interface. Nachemson[29] has suggested that some of the stability of the spine in antigravity postures is due to the activity of the psoas major muscles, and may in fact partially account for the recorded intradiscal pressures with various postures.

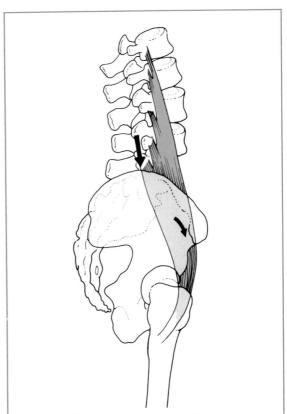

Figure 3–27. Lateral view depicting an inferior and posterior moment imparted to the superior lateral pubic ramus as a result of the contraction of the iliopsoas muscle complex in a closed kinetic chain. This contraction results in an anterior torsion of the ilium and an extension force imparted to the lumbosacral zygapophyseal joints.

ground and contraction of the iliacus muscle occurs, the resultant force to the ilium produces an anterior torsion of the ilium and extension of the lumbosacral zygapophyseal joints (Fig. 3–27). Anterior torsion of the ilium represents a forward and downward movement of the anterior superior iliac spines. Extension to the lumbosacral joints can also occur as a result of the anterior pelvic rotation, which causes the superior articular process of S1 to move up on the inferior articular process of the L5 vertebrae.

If there is decreased length of the muscle owing to adaptive shortening, or if there is increased efferent neural input into the muscle, then a downwardly tilted or anteriorly rotated position of the complete pelvis results. This increases the compressive load on the lumbar zygapophyseal joints (see Chapter 4).

It is interesting to note that the psoas major muscle is more consistently active than other trunk muscles when a person assumes a variety of positions. When the importance of stability of the lumbar spine rather than actual movement is considered, the potential stabilization role of the psoas major muscle becomes extremely important. This is especially true when analyzing the guy wire action of the psoas muscle as it works with the deep portion of the erector spinae, multifidus, and quadratus lumborum muscles for stability in the sagittal, frontal, and horizontal planes. The guy wire stabilization concept, coupled with the compression of the vertebral bodies in the weight-bearing postures, results in securing the interlocking assembly of the lower lumbar articulations. This in turn renders the lumbar joints more resistant to various forces. In both stabilization and movement roles the iliopsoas muscle presumably contracts to counterbalance the forces of the posterior lumbar muscles, creating equilibrium. The balance assures nondestructive force attenuation of the lumbar vertebral tissues.

We seldom lift or bend in a pure sagittal plane while performing activities of daily living. Instead, we lift with varying amounts of rotation and side bending. It is the coordinated concentric and eccentric contractions of the psoas major and other related lumbopelvic muscles that directly control the weight-bearing properties of the lumbar spine during this asymmetrical motion.

Depending on the side to which the spine is laterally bent and rotated, both psoas major muscles must respond appropriately. Gracovetsky and Farfan[15] present a mathematical model describing the function of the psoas major muscle in lifting and walking. The iliopsoas muscle appears to have a significant function in the three cardinal planes of motion, thus the importance of adequate strength and coordination of the iliopsoas muscle in stabilization and movement of the lumbar spine.

A consideration of the adequacy of muscle length is equally important. When the normal postural positions of the adult are analyzed, it is apparent that a sitting position is common in both work and rest. The effect of these prolonged postures might be to adaptively shorten the iliopsoas muscle. When the person now assumes the upright position, or if the hip is placed in hyperextension, the lumbar spine is pulled forward and downward, which causes

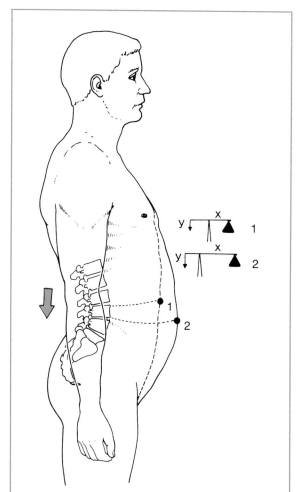

Figure 3–28. A pendulous abdomen renders the lumbar spine vulnerable to increased weight-bearing demands. In the example of the abdomen (1) the distance from the center of the spine and the abdominal wall is X, and the muscle force to counterbalance the lever arm is Y. In example (2), the distance from the center of the spine and the abdominal wall is X+ and the muscle force to counteract the lever arm is Y+. This increased muscular force results in elevated lumbar vertebral weight-bearing. (Adapted from White AA, Panjabi MM: Clinical Biomechanics of the Spine. J.B. Lippincott, Philadelphia, 1978.)

an extension and compression moment to the lumbar zygapophyseal joints. Weight-bearing demands of all of the lumbar tissues, in this example, are now being loaded in the upper portion of the optimal loading zone (see Chapter 1). By virtue of the posterior and inferior resultant forces of the iliopsoas at the lateral aspect of the superior ramus of the pubis, the lumbar spine must move forward and downward toward the lesser trochanters as the lower extremities are placed under the body.

If this posture is further compounded by a pendulous abdomen, it is readily apparent that the unbalanced forces result in faulty and potentially injurious postural mechanics. In order to maintain the upright posture and counterbalance the pendulous abdomen, the person must further extend the trunk, increasing the weight-bearing demands on the lumbar tissues under compression (Fig. 3–28). Posterior lumbar tissues, such as the zygapophyseal joints, may be the source of pain, but the cause is probably altered postural mechanics.

The function of the psoas major muscle must, therefore, be looked at in terms of strength, coordination, and adequate length. Because it is strategically placed, it has numerous control functions related to lumbar spine motions, and shortness or altered contraction patterns of the muscle jeopardize the normal biomechanical relation between the intervertebral discs and zygapophyseal joints.

THE ABDOMINAL WALL

The vertebrae, intervertebral disc, zygapophyseal joints, and intervening soft tissues of the vertebral column are subjected to large forces during work, athletics, and daily activities. In its simplest description, the spine can be considered to be an elastic rod that responds in different ways to forces placed on it.

The abdominal wall musculature has been extensively studied by both experiment and mathematical modeling.[1,14,28,31,37,40] Various roles have been attributed to the musculature related to the spine, but most authorities agree that this muscle group is important in offering stability to the vertebral column. The abdominal wall consists of the external abdominal oblique, internal abdominal oblique, transversus abdominis, and rectus abdominis muscles, and the fascial contributions of these muscles form the rectus sheath.

The external abdominal oblique muscle originates by way of fleshy digitations to the last eight ribs and extends inferiorly to insert into the iliac crest, and inferiorly and medially to blend with the abdominal aponeurosis and linea alba. It is the largest and most superficial anterolateral muscle.[16] Between the anterior superior iliac spine and pubic tubercle it forms a thick, inrolled band known as the inguinal ligament.

The internal abdominal oblique muscle is deep to the external abdominal oblique muscle. This muscle is attached to the lateral half of the inguinal ligament, the iliac crest, and the inferior portion of the lateral raphe of the thoracolumbar fascia. From these attachments the muscle extends superiorly and medially to insert into the cartilaginous border of the last three or four ribs, the abdominal aponeurosis, and the linea alba.

Although most of the fibers of the internal abdominal oblique muscle attach to the iliac crest, the posterior fibers arise from the fused layers of the thoracolumbar fascia. In some people the attachment of the internal abdominal oblique muscle is solely to the iliac crest, whereas in others it may arise entirely from the fusion of the fascial layers at the lateral border of the erector spinae muscles.[4]

The orientation of the muscle fibers of both the external and internal abdominal oblique muscles helps to predict their function during contraction. The inferior and medial direction of the fibers of the external abdominal oblique muscle are positioned to posteriorly rotate the pelvis or check the downward and forward motion of the pelvis.[22] The superior and medial fibers of the internal abdominal oblique muscle are best positioned to flex the trunk (Fig. 3–29A and B).

The transversus abdominis muscle is located deep to the internal abdominal oblique muscle. It is attached to the lateral one third of the inguinal ligament, the inner lip of the iliac crest, and the thoracolumbar fascia in a common attachment shared by the internal abdominal

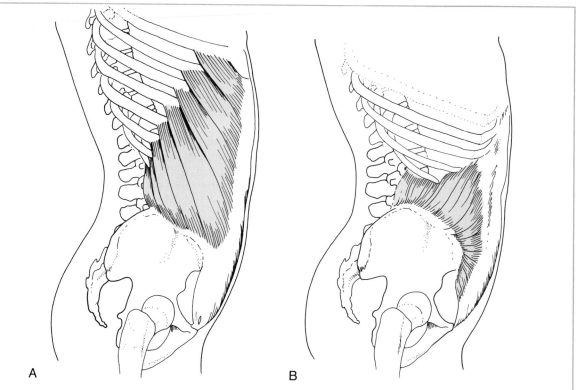

Figure 3–29. *A*, Inferior and medial direction of the external oblique muscles are best positioned to check the downward and forward motion of the pelvis, i.e., check anterior torsion of the ilium and extension of lumbar zygapophyseal joints. *B*, Superior and medial direction of the internal oblique muscles are best positioned to flex the trunk. Together these abdominal oblique muscles form a major balance or check to lumbar weight-bearing.

oblique. The fiber direction is more horizontal than that of the internal oblique muscle as it runs to attach to the abdominal aponeurosis and the linea alba.

The last division of the abdominal wall is the rectus abdominis muscle. This muscle extends vertically from the pubic tubercles to attach to the lower rib cage on either side of the sternum. The rectus abdominis muscle is a long, straplike muscle that is divided by intermuscular connective tissue bands. These muscles lie on either side of the linea alba and are positioned to flex the trunk as well as to help contain the abdominal contents.

The rectus abdominis muscle is surrounded by its own fascial layer (the rectus sheath),

formed by the individual fascial contributions of the transversus abdominis, external oblique, and internal oblique muscles as they converge toward the linea alba (Fig. 3–30). Above the umbilicus the external oblique muscle sends its aponeurosis anterior to the rectus. The aponeurosis of the internal abdominal oblique muscle splits at the lateral border of the rectus abdominis, and the aponeurosis passes anterior and posterior to it. The aponeurosis of the transversus abdominis muscle travels behind the rectus abdominis muscle.

Below the umbilicus all three lateral abdominal muscles pass aponeurotic expansions anterior to the rectus abdominis muscle. There is no specific explanation for this anatomical

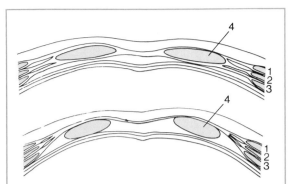

Figure 3–30. Cross section of the abdominal wall showing the relation between the abdominal aponeurosis and the rectus abdominis muscle above and below the umbilicus. *Above the umbilicus* the aponeurosis of the external oblique muscle (1) and one half of the internal oblique muscle (2) travel in front of the rectus abdominis muscle (4), and the other half of the aponeurosis of the internal oblique muscle and the transversus abdominis muscle (3) travel behind the rectus abdominis muscle (4). *Below the umbilicus* the aponeurosis from all three abdominal muscles (1, 2, 3) travel in front of the rectus abdominis muscle (4). The functional significance is probably an increased stability below the umbilicus to correspond to the angle change at the L4 and L5 lumbar segments.

variation, but it is logical to conclude that below the umbilicus the added aponeurosis in front of the rectus offers additional support for this region. The extra fascial support is perhaps a response to the forces generated from the lordotic angle at the corresponding level in the lumbar spine (i.e., the L4–L5 and L5–S1 region). In this region of the lumbar spine the rate of curvature is greater than the rate of curvature for the upper lumbar spine. Accompanying this skeletal change is the increased inferiorly and anteriorly directed force of the abdominal contents, which helps to create the need for the additional connective tissue support.

There are many theories about the role of the abdominal muscles with regard to supporting the spine. Morris and coworkers[28] suggested that the abdominal muscles, working with the pelvic floor, diaphragm, and epiglottis, helped to convert the thoracic and abdominal chambers that are filled with air and semisolid contents into rigid cylinders. These cylinders hypothetically helped to unload the spine by actually transmitting part of the forces applied. The cavities become pressurized cylinders that help to absorb forces.

Gracovetsky and Farfan[14] have taken this concept of increased intra-abdominal pressure one step further. Rather than consider that the intra-abdominal pressure unloads the spine, they suggest that the oblique direction of the abdominal musculature contracts around a pressurized cylinder instead of simply contracting and collapsing toward the center. They theorize that the internal oblique and transversus abdominis muscles exert a lateral and posteriorly directed pull to their attachment at the lateral raphe of the thoracolumbar fascia. As previously described, the lateral raphe lies posterior and lateral to the transverse process of the vertebrae.

Tesh and associates[40] explain that the transversus abdominis muscle and the internal abdominal oblique muscle attach by way of the middle layer of the thoracolumbar fascia in a direct line to the transverse process, and consequently contribute to the stability of the spine by a laterally directed pull on the vertebrae. The controlled contraction of the abdominal wall would minimize lumbar movement in the frontal and horizontal planes. Likewise, the attachment of the external oblique to the ribs and the iliac crest provides efficient leverage, relative to the lumbopelvic joints, to offer a resistance to axial rotation and lateral motions.

Rather than considering the abdominal muscles as flexors and rotators of the trunk—which they certainly have the capability to do—their function may be best viewed as antirotators and antilateral flexors. The trunk must be stabilized against excessive rotation forces that accompany upper and lower extremity motion.

The abdominal wall musculature works synergistically with other muscles during functional activities, presumably to assist with movement as well as stabilization functions. For example, in lifting, muscles like the gluteus maximus, quadriceps, and spinal extensors are positioned to provide the necessary forces to return to the upright position. The abdominal oblique muscles are oriented to minimize excessive motions of the lumbopelvic region in the horizontal and frontal planes. These two planes are actually linked because the lumbar spine is a curved column. In any curved column lateral bending causes an axial rotation, and conversely, an axial rotation causes lateral bending.

Because of their attachments to the rib cage and the pelvis, the abdominal muscles are effective rotators of the spine. However, there is only a small degree of rotary motion available at each lumbar zygapophyseal joint; consequently the abdominal oblique muscles presumably offer stabilization in the horizontal plane by controlling rotary forces that reach the lumbopelvic tissues and by minimizing the chance of torsional injuries. As mentioned earlier, the degree of curvature in the lower lumbar spine is greater than that in the upper lumbar spine. This is of interest because the majority of zygapophyseal joint and disc degeneration problems are usually greater in the lower lumbar region. Many activities require motion of the lumbar spine. Recognizing that only small amounts of lateral bend or axial rotation cause obligatory coupled motion, a muscular design that minimizes these forces that reach the lower lumbar spine appears critical.

The muscular design of the abdominal wall reemphasizes the concept of dynamic stabilization and the underlying role of the central nervous system. It is logical to conclude that with a strong and functionally trained or neuromuscularly coordinated abdominal wall, the ability to keep destructive forces away from the lumbopelvic tissues is enhanced. As previously emphasized, this is accomplished by directing the forces of weight-bearing and movement through the proper tissues and by keeping the weight-bearing line in check (see Chapter 6).

Abdominal wall musculature without adequate endurance, strength, and coordination appears more likely to permit other lumbar-stabilizing and weight-bearing tissues to be taken past their physiologic limit, such as excessive tensile forces on the annulus or excessive compressive forces on the zygapophyseal joints. Thus the musculature of the abdominal wall plays a considerable role in the maintenance of a healthy lumbar spine.

MUSCULATURE OF THE HIP

The iliopsoas muscles have been previously described with the muscles of the lumbar spine, since the psoas major has significant attachments to the lumbar spine. A brief review of the remaining musculature of the hip is necessary to gain a more thorough understanding of lumbopelvic mechanics.

There are 29 muscles that originate or insert into the pelvis. Twenty of these muscles link the pelvis with the femur, and the remainder link the pelvis with the spine. This implies that significant forces can be generated through the pelvis and subsequently into the lumbar spine by various combinations of hip muscle activity. It is not just the muscles above the pelvis (lumbar spine and abdominal wall musculature), but also the muscles from below (muscles of the hip joint) that work synergistically to assure proper attenuation of forces through the lumbar spine.

Anterior Thigh Musculature Functioning at the Hip

The sartorius and rectus femoris muscles attach to the anterior pelvis and proceed inferiorly to cross the knee joint. These muscles have well-recognized actions at the hip and knee joints, but they can also play a role in the generation of forces to the pelvis (Fig. 3–31). For example, if either has increased tension owing to an increased efferent motor response, or tightness owing to adaptive shortening, an increased anterior moment to the ilium can result as tension in the muscle increases.

As previously mentioned, this anterior movement to the ilium can increase the extension forces to the tissues of the lumbar spine. These muscles, coupled with a tight iliopsoas muscle and a tight hip joint capsule on the ipsilateral side, render the lumbopelvic articulations vulnerable to injury. Because the sagittal plane mechanics of the lumbopelvic tissue are now altered, adaptive changes to accommodate new tissue stresses are inevitable. The L5–S1 zygapophyseal joints, for example, must endure increased vertical forces. Recognition of the influence of the sartorius and rectus fe-

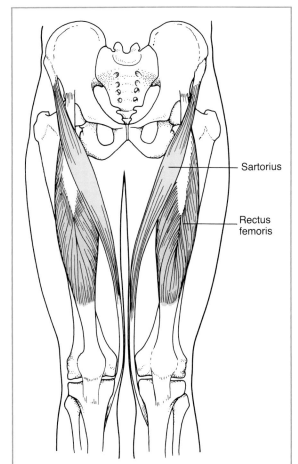

Figure 3–31. The relation of the rectus femoris muscle (1) and the sartorius muscle (2) to the lumbopelvic region. Contraction of these muscles impart forces to the pelvis and hip joint that affect weight-bearing of the lumbopelvic region.

moris muscles on sagittal plane mechanics warrants their attention during lumbopelvic evaluation.

Medial Thigh Musculature Functioning at the Hip

The pectineus, adductor brevis, adductor longus, anterior aspect of the adductor magnus, and gracilis muscles attach to the pubic and ischial rami, and extend inferiorly and laterally to attach to the femur. These muscles are considered to be adductors and rotators of the femur in the open kinetic chain. The first three muscles are also femoral flexors.

However, when the foot is fixed on the ground, contraction of these muscles imparts a force to the pelvis that influences the frontal and sagittal plane positions of the lumbopelvic unit. This ultimately affects the weight-bearing positions of the lumbar spine and the sacroiliac and hip joints. Note how these muscles must work with the quadratus lumborum and psoas major muscles to control the frontal plane position of the spine and pelvis (Fig. 3–32). These muscles also impart an anterior rotational force to the pelvis by virtue of their attachments to it. This force can be due to the extended position of the femur or to the contraction of these muscles when the femur is fixed.

The functions of these muscles when the opposite limb is in swing phase of gait should be considered. They work with the abductors on the same side to create a weight-bearing posture of the hip joint to assure the proper transference of forces. These muscle groups probably contract together not only to balance the pelvis and stabilize the joints of the spine, but also to properly secure the acetabulum onto the femoral head. This demonstrates the importance of evaluating function in the weight-bearing position.

Lateral Thigh Musculature Functioning at the Hip

The muscles of the lateral thigh include the gluteus medius and minimis and the tensor fascia latae (Fig. 3–33). They play an important role in the frontal plane stability of the lumbopelvic unit. Therefore, it is important that they work in a synergistic manner with the medial thigh muscles and lateral trunk muscles to assure that nondestructive weight-bearing patterns occur.

For example, if there is a difference in strength of the right and left hip abductor muscles, then the amount of frontal plane motion during stance phase of gait varies. One side of the pelvis drops further than the other because of the inability of the hip abductors to stabilize

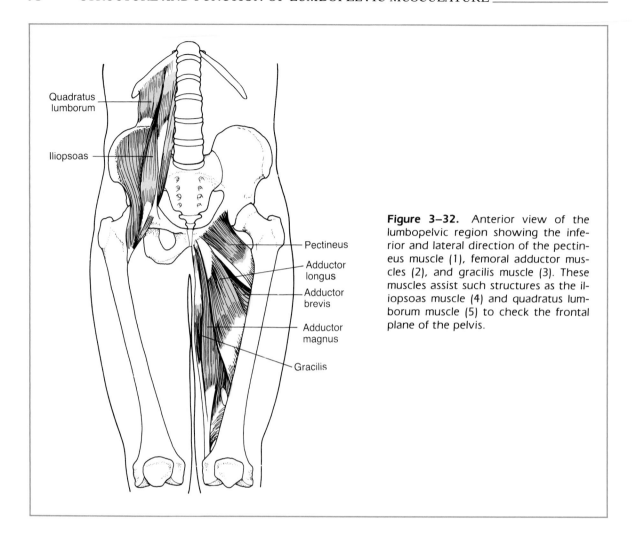

Quadratus lumborum

Iliopsoas

Pectineus

Adductor longus

Adductor brevis

Adductor magnus

Gracilis

Figure 3–32. Anterior view of the lumbopelvic region showing the inferior and lateral direction of the pectineus muscle (1), femoral adductor muscles (2), and gracilis muscle (3). These muscles assist such structures as the iliopsoas muscle (4) and quadratus lumborum muscle (5) to check the frontal plane of the pelvis.

the pelvis. Taken one step further, this excessive frontal plane motion of the pelvis can also result in excessive compressive forces to the lumbar spine, since lateral bending and rotation are coupled motions.

Because the weight-bearing line is shifted to either side owing to hip abductor weakness, the forces on the femoral head are also altered. In the example above the right femur is now relatively adducted when compared with the left. The compressive force on the right femoral head is now different from the compressive force on the left femoral head. Friberg[13] has noted that a relatively adducted femur leaves the lower extremity in a varus position. The varus position also increases compressive forces to the lateral aspect of the greater trochanter owing to the stretched lateral hip musculature (Fig. 3–34A and B). This compressive force, if prolonged or excessive, may result in inflammation to the bursa that lies beneath the hip abductor tendon. Greater trochanteric bursitis may be a result of altered frontal plane biomechanics. Treatment of the irritated bursa tissue is most successful when the forces that are responsible for its irritation are minimized.

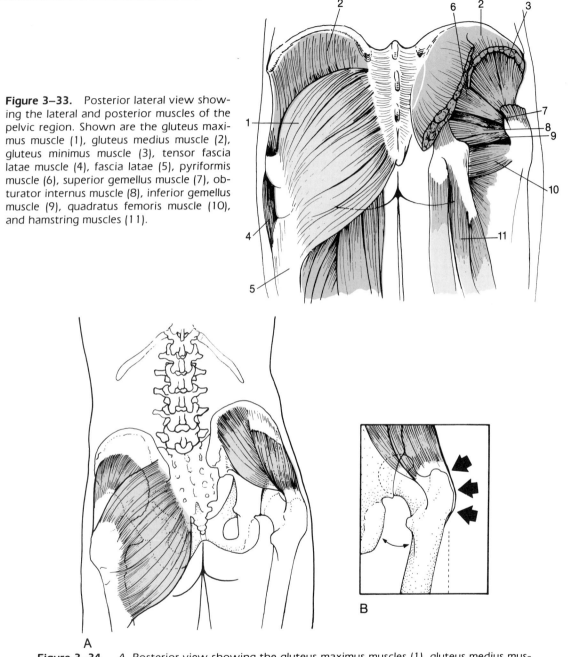

Figure 3–33. Posterior lateral view showing the lateral and posterior muscles of the pelvic region. Shown are the gluteus maximus muscle (1), gluteus medius muscle (2), gluteus minimus muscle (3), tensor fascia latae muscle (4), fascia latae (5), pyriformis muscle (6), superior gemellus muscle (7), obturator internus muscle (8), inferior gemellus muscle (9), quadratus femoris muscle (10), and hamstring muscles (11).

Figure 3–34. *A,* Posterior view showing the gluteus maximus muscles (1), gluteus medius muscles (2), and the underlying gluteus minimus muscles as they insert into the greater trochanter of the femur. The greater trochanteric bursae lies under this tendinous attachment and over the greater trochanter. *B,* Expanded view: In an example of a left frontal plane asymmetry (sacral tilt to the left), the right femur adopts an adducted position, increasing the compressive force to the greater trochanteric bursae.

Posterior Thigh Musculature Functioning at the Hip

The posterior thigh muscles combine to form a large and powerful muscle group composed of the gluteus maximus and hamstring muscles. In addition, the deep rotator muscles of the hip, such as the obturator internus and externus, superior and inferior gemelli, quadratus femoris, and piriformis, work in concert with the gluteus maximus and hamstring muscles. These muscles all have the potential to exert forces on the lumbopelvic region because of their pelvic and sacral attachments. As pointed out earlier, the force of the muscle contraction is readily transmitted to the pelvis when the femur or foot becomes fixed and a closed kinetic chain is established.

These muscles influence sagittal plane mechanics, especially by exerting a posterior rotary moment on the pelvis. This action results in flexion of the lumbosacral region (Fig. 3–35).

The deep lateral rotators are probably not strong prime movers, especially in the closed kinetic chain, yet they presumably assist in stabilizing the femoral head in the acetabulum.

The posterior thigh muscles are important in controlling many motions of the pelvis. It must be recognized, however, that the contraction of these prime movers can and probably does exert large forces to the lumbopelvic articulations by virtue of their size and anatomical position. For example, in forward bending these posterior muscles contract eccentrically to control the pelvis so that smooth trunk flexion can occur. Once the movement reaches the pelvis, there is an anterior motion around the hip joints and the knees most often bend. Returning from the forward bending position requires a stabilizing contraction at the pelvis so that the trunk musculature can have a solid base from which to contract. As the motion continues, these posterior muscles concentrically contract to posteriorly rotate the pelvis to complete the movement.

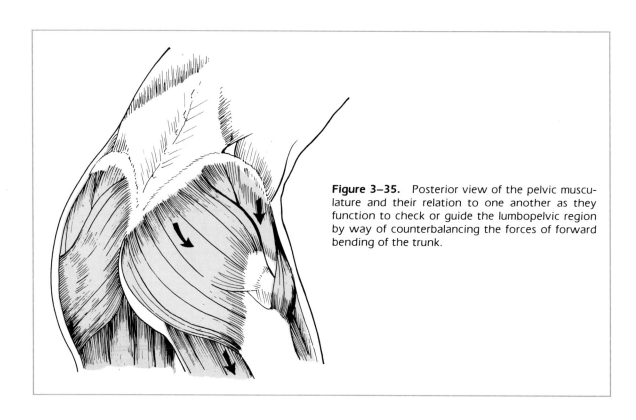

Figure 3–35. Posterior view of the pelvic musculature and their relation to one another as they function to check or guide the lumbopelvic region by way of counterbalancing the forces of forward bending of the trunk.

SUMMARY

The musculature of the lumbopelvic region is designed to initiate and control multiplanar movements and to assist in the attenuation of forces reaching the lumbopelvic region. The central nervous system ultimately controls the motor behavior of these tissues. As in the extremities, a balance of muscle strength, neuromuscular coordination, and tissue length must be maintained in order to avoid injury. Although the intervertebral discs are often considered to be shock absorbers for the spine, it is actually the musculature that is responsible for shock absorption.[18] The physiology of passive and active muscle tension is therefore an important consideration.

As the musculoskeletal tissues adaptively change with age, and as the body heals from previous injuries, the force absorption and transferral capabilities of this hub of weight-bearing diminish. Painful mechanical syndromes often result. The lumbopelvic musculature is detailed not only to assist the reader in functional assessment, but also to provide a foundation from which to build therapeutic exercise programs. Without an appreciation of the structure and function of the lumbopelvic musculature, successful long-term management and prevention programs are difficult to achieve.

REFERENCES

1. Bankoff ADP, Furlani J: Electromyographic study of the rectus abdominis and external oblique muscles during exercises. Electromyogr Clin Neurophysiol 24:501, 1984.
2. Bigland-Ritchie B: Muscle fatigue and the influence of changing neural drive. Symposium on Exercise: Physiology and Clinical Application. Clin Chest Med 5:21, 1984.
3. Bogduk N: A reappraisal of the anatomy of the human erector spinae. J Anat 131:525, 1980.
4. Bogduk N, Macintosh JE: The applied anatomy of the thoracolumbar fascia. Spine 9:164, 1984.
5. Bogduk N, Twomey LT: Clinical Anatomy of the Lumbar Spine. London, Churchill Livingstone, 1987.
6. Bustami FMF: A new description of the lumbar erector spinae in man. J Anat 144:81, 1986.
7. Carew TJ, Ghez C: Muscles and muscle receptors. In Kandel ER, Schwartz JS (eds): Principles of Neural Science, 2nd ed. New York, Elsevier, 1985, p. 443.
8. Carr D, Gilbertson L, Frymoyer J, et al: Lumbar paraspinal compartment syndrome: A case report with physiologic and anatomic studies. Spine 10:816, 1985.
9. Donisch EW, Basmajian JV: Electromyography of deep back muscles in man. Am J Anat 133:25, 1972.
10. Farfan HF: Mechanical Disorders of the Lowback. Philadelphia, Lea & Febiger, 1973.
11. Farfan HF: Muscular mechanism of the lumbar spine and the position of power and efficiency. Orthop Clin North Am 6:135, 1975.
12. Floyd WF, Silver PHS: The function of erector spine muscles in certain movements and postures in man. J Physiol 129:184, 1955.
13. Friberg O: Clinical symptoms and biomechanics of lumbar spine and hip joint in leg length inequality. Spine 8:643, 1983.
14. Gracovetsky S, Farfan HF, Helleur C: The abdominal mechanism. Spine 10:317, 1985.
15. Gracovetsky S, Farfan H: The optimum spine. Spine 11:543, 1986.
16. Warwick R, Williams P (eds): Gray's Anatomy, 35th ed. London, Longmans, 1980.
17. Hollinshead WH, Rosse C: The vertebral column. In Textbook of Human Anatomy, 4th ed, p. 285. Philadelphia, Harper & Row, 1985.
18. Hukins DWL: Disc structure and function. In Ghosh P (ed): The Biology of the Intervertebral Disc, vol I. Boca Raton, Fla, CRC Press, 1988, p. 1.
19. Huxley HE, Hanson J: The structure and function of muscle. vol I, Bourne GH (ed), New York, Academic Press, 1960.
20. Kandel ER: Factors controlling transmitter release. In Kandel ER, Swartz JH (eds): Principles of Neurosciences. New York, Elsevier, 1985, p. 120.
21. Kapandji IA: The Physiology of the Joints, vol 3. Edinburgh, Churchill Livingstone, 1974.
22. Kendall F, McCreary EK: Muscles: Testing and Function, 3rd ed. Baltimore, Williams & Wilkins, 1983.
23. Kippers V, Parker AW: Posture related to myoelectric silence of erector spinae during trunk flexion. Spine 9:740, 1984.
24. Luk KDK, Ho HC, Leong JCY: The iliolumbar ligament: A study of its anatomy, development, and clinical significance. J Bone Joint Surg 68:197, 1986.
25. McArdle WD, Katch FI, Katch VL: Skeletal muscle: Structure and function. In Exercise Physiology: Energy, Nutrition, and Human Performance, p. 289. Philadelphia, Lea & Febiger, 1986.
26. McGill SM, Norman RW: Partitioning of the L4–L5 dynamic moment into disc, ligamentous, and muscular components during lifting. Spine 11:566, 1986.
27. Morris JM, Benner G, Lucas DB: An electromyographic study of the intrinsic muscles of the back in man. J Anat 96:509, 1962.
28. Morris JM, Lucas DB, Bresler B: The role of the trunk in stability of the spine. J Bone Joint Surg 43A:327, 1961.
29. Nachemson A: Electromyographic studies of the ver-

tebral portion of the psoas muscle. Acta Orthop Scand 37:177, 1966.

30. Nordin M, Frankel VH: Biomechanics of tendons and ligaments. In Frankel VH, Nordin M: Basic Biomechanics of the Skeletal System. Philadelphia, Lea & Febiger, 1989, p. 59.

31. Ortengren R, Andersson GBJ: Electromyographic studies of trunk muscles with special reference to the functional anatomy of the lumbar spine. Spine 2:44, 1977.

32. Paris SV: Anatomy as related to function and pain. Orthop Clin North Am 14:475, 1983.

33. Pauly JE: An electromyographic analysis of certain movements and exercises in some deep back muscles. Anat Rec 155:223, 1966.

34. Peck D, Nicholls PJ, Beard C, Allen JR: Are there compartment syndromes in some patients with idiopathic back pain. Spine 11:468, 1986.

35. Porterfield JA: Dynamic stabilization of the trunk. J Orthop Sports Phys Ther 6:271, 1985.

36. Schultz A, Anderson GBJ, Ortengren R, et al: Analysis and quantitative myoelectric measurements of loads on the lumbar spine when holding weights in standing postures. Spine 7:390, 1982.

37. Seroussi RE, Pope MH: The relationship between trunk muscle electromyography and lifting movements in the sagittal and frontal planes. J Biomech 20:135, 1987.

38. Sirca A, Kostevc V: The fibre type composition of thoracic and lumbar paravertebral muscles in man. J Anat 141:131, 1985.

39. Sullivan MS: Back support mechanisms during manual lifting. Phys Ther 69:38, 1989.

40. Tesh KM, Dunn JS, Evans JH: The abdominal muscles and vertebral stability. Spine 12:501, 1987.

41. Valencia FP, Munro RR: An electromyographic study of the lumbar multifidus in man. Electromyogr Clin Neurophysiol 25:205, 1985.

42. Vander AJ, Sherman JH, Luciano DS: Biological control systems: Muscle. In Human Physiology: The Mechanism of Body Function. New York, McGraw-Hill, 1976, p. 34.

43. Wolf SL, Basmajian JV, Russe CTC, Kutner M: Normative data on low back mobility and activity levels. Am J Phys Med 58:217, 1979.

44. Woo SL-Y, Buckwalter JA: Injury and Repair of the Musculoskeletal Soft Tissues. Park Ridge, Ill, American Academy of Orthopedic Surgeons, 1988.

4

ARTICULATIONS OF THE LUMBOPELVIC REGION

A separate chapter regarding the articulations of the lumbopelvic region is necessary in order to appropriately detail their structure and function. A great deal of experimental study and observation by engineers, anatomists, and orthopedic specialists regarding these joints have been documented in the literature, and these investigations have helped to form the rationale for many orthopedic therapeutic interventions.

As with all articulations of the musculoskeletal system, the interplay between the articulating components and their connective tissue stabilizers and associated muscles, and, more important, the efficiency by which smooth movement occurs, are impossible to completely comprehend. However, studies of the articulations have allowed for speculation as to the mechanical function of the joints, and this in turn has led to various approaches toward evaluation and treatment.

Because low back pain remains a major concern to society in terms of cost, work loss, and suffering, the articulations of this area have been subject to a great deal of experimental study. In some regards the articulations have been detailed more extensively than the surrounding muscular system, which is unfortunate because of the important role muscles play in the overall function of the lumbopelvic region. The articulations and related soft tissues work together in the attenuation of forces. It is the purpose of this chapter to describe the anatomy and function of the various articula-

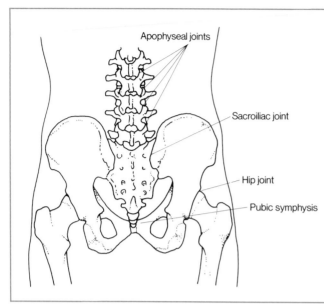

Apophyseal joints

Sacroiliac joint

Hip joint

Pubic symphysis

Figure 4–1. A posterior view of the lumbopelvic region emphasizing the inferior articulating process of the vertebra above to the superior articulating process of the vertebra below. This view shows the articulations and bony structures of the lumbopelvic region.

tions of the lumbopelvic region in order to better understand their synergistic relationship with one another and the neuromuscular systems.

The articulations that will be discussed include the L4-L5 and lumbosacral (L5-S1) zygapophysial joints, intervertebral discs (specific mention will be made of the intervertebral discs between the fourth and fifth lumbar vertebrae, and between the fifth lumbar vertebra and sacrum), sacroiliac joints, symphysis pubis, and hips (Fig. 4–1). These articulations define the lumbopelvic articulations for the purposes of this text, and are chosen to detail because of the contribution each makes to the transference of trunk and ground forces.

THE ZYGAPOPHYSEAL JOINTS AS A COMPONENT OF THE FUNCTIONAL UNIT

It should be stated from the onset that to consider the zygapophyseal joints separate from the intervertebral disc–vertebral body interface disregards the true movement pattern of the lumbar spine. Forces that occur because of

weight-bearing, movement, or muscle contraction do not selectively affect the zygapophyseal joints, but ultimately all tissues of the spine. The zygapophyseal joints, intervertebral disc, and surrounding tissues work together as a functional unit that allows for these forces to be transferred through the lumbar spine.

Because of this smooth interplay between all tissues of the lumbar spine, an injury to the zygapophyseal joints potentially alters the function of surrounding tissues. Therefore, caution must be taken in analyzing the function of these joints. The intervertebral "joint" in the lumbar spine is actually the combined structures of the intervertebral disc–vertebral body interface and the zygapophyseal joints with the surrounding ligamentous and muscular tissue.

To emphasize this relationship between the zygapophyseal joint and the intervertebral disc, Panjabi and colleagues[69] used the terminology "functional spinal unit" to refer to the smallest segment from which to analyze segmental mechanics. They suggest that disc injury has the effect of altering spinal kinematics above and below that level, which in turn leads to asymmetrical movements and loading at the lumbar zygapophyseal joints (Fig. 4–2).

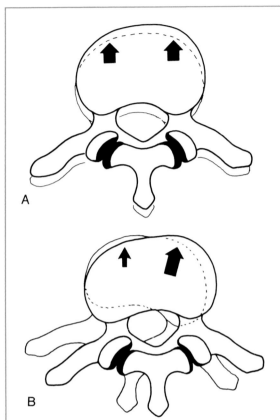

Figure 4–2. *A,* Transverse section of a functional spinal unit showing the functional relation with an anterior shear of the top vertebra on the bottom vertebra. This motion is best checked by the apophyseal joint and the intervertebral disc. *B,* With an injury to the intervertebral disc the kinematics of the functional segmental unit is altered. In this example, as the top vertebra begins to shear anterior, as in *A,* the intervertebral disc does not respond to the impending stress, thus increasing the load to the right apophyseal joint and rendering it vulnerable to overload.

These abnormal, asymmetrical forces produce functional adaptation that is followed by structural adaptation. In the zygapophyseal joints the response of the facets (which are the articulating surfaces of the zygapophyseal joints) to abnormal loading patterns or direct injury might be cartilage degeneration, facet atrophy, and, if excessive forces are maintained over a long period, bony adaption in the

form of sclerosis or spurring.[87,103] The changes in structure alter joint function, which in turn alters intervertebral disc mechanics. Likewise, intervertebral disc injury alters the manner in which the zygapophyseal joints function. This helps to underscore the significance of the synergistic roles played by these structures in the attenuation of forces.

REGIONAL ANATOMY OF THE ZYGAPOPHYSEAL JOINTS

The zygapophyseal joints of the lumbar spine are synovial joints formed by the articulation between the inferior articular process of one vertebra and the superior articular process of the vertebra immediately below. In the lumbar spine the inferior articular process is medial to the superior articular process (Fig. 4–3).

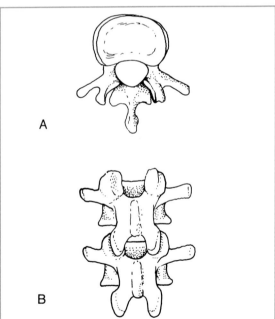

Figure 4–3. *A,* Transverse view of the relation of the inferior articulating process of the vertebra above, which is medial to the superior articulating process of the vertebra below. *B,* Posterior view of the vertebral segment emphasizing the medial relation of the inferior articulating process to the superior articulating process.

These joints feature the elements typical of synovial joints, including articular cartilage, synovial lining, synovial fluid, and a joint capsule.

Each articular process is covered with hyaline cartilage with a thickness typically ranging from 2 to 4 mm.[60,61] This thickness of the cartilage contributes to methods of force acceptance in these lumbar joints. For example, when forces are applied that result in compression of these joint surfaces, the approximation results in water being squeezed out of the hyaline cartilage. When the compressive forces are removed, fluid seeps back into the hyaline cartilage. Although this behavior typifies the normal response of the healthy articular cartilage of any synovial joint to compressive forces, it is mentioned in reference to the zygapophyseal joints in order to emphasize that they, too, have a role in weight-bearing. Some of these weight-bearing functions also occur when the lumbar spine assumes various postures. Cartilage deformation followed by the restoration of thickness is, therefore, important not only for nutritive functions, but also in force transference.

The orientation of the lumbar joint surfaces (the facet planes) is not simple, flat planar surfaces, as implied in some mechanical models. The articular cartilage cover, plus the shape of the bony process itself, gives the zygapophyseal joints more of a compound surface, that is, a surface that faces in more than one plane. There is often a convex–concave orientation, with the inferior articular process forming the convex partner and the superior process forming the concave one.

The concavity of the superior articular process is also functionally deepened by the posterior aspect of the ligamentum flavum (Fig. 4–4). The inferior articular process can ride on the posterolateral surface of the ligamentum flavum during movement. Some cadaver specimens show the development of fibrous cartilage on this corner of the ligamentum flavum, perhaps typifying the response of the ligament to the various stresses placed on it.

The articulations between the inferior and superior articular processes of adjacent lumbar vertebrae are not true ball-and-socket articulations, but rather a structural arrangement

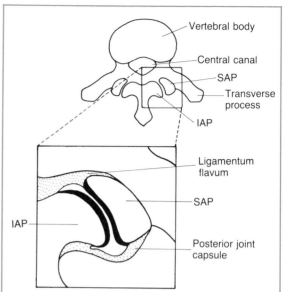

Figure 4–4. *Transverse view of the vertebral segment emphasizing the convexity of the inferior articulating process (IAP) and the concavity of the superior articulating process (SAP) of the right apophyseal articulation. Note the deepening of the concavity of the SAP by the ligamentum flavum.*

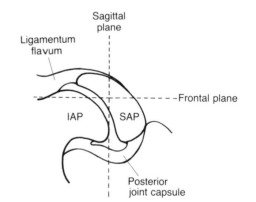

Figure 4–5. *Close-up of transverse section of a right apophyseal joint revealing the two planes (sagittal and frontal planes) made up by the articulations of the IAP and SAP.*

that allows the portions of the individual facet of the zygapophyseal joint to simultaneously face in at least two planes. Two obvious planes of alignment seen with facet orientation of the L4-L5 and lumbosacral articulations are the frontal and sagittal (Fig. 4–5). The importance of these planes is addressed when function is discussed, but it is important to note that there are varying degrees of sagittal and frontal plane orientation at all levels of the lumbar spine. There is also asymmetry between two sides of the same vertebra. These variations contribute to the differences between the joints of the upper and lower lumbar spine.[21,54,97]

THE LIGAMENTUM FLAVUM AND THE APOPHYSEAL JOINT CAPSULE

If the concave surface of the superior articular facet is followed medially, the posterolateral aspect of the ligamentum flavum is reached. As mentioned already, this ligament further increases the concavity of the superior articular surface, and the posterior aspect of the ligamentum can function as an articular surface to the inferior facet.

The ligamentum flavum increases the surface area that is oriented in the frontal plane of the zygapophyseal joint. Engagement by the two articulating partners of the joint occurs when the inferior articulating process of the vertebra above shears forward (anterior shear of the superior vertebra) on the vertebra below. This anterior shear force is greatest at the lower lumbar levels (L4-L5 and L5-S1) because the curve of the lower lumbar spine is more pronounced than the curve in the upper lumbar spine (Fig. 4–6). The anterior shear force is also greater in the standing position than in the sitting position because of the different degree of lordosis that results with the two postures.

Therefore, the erect posture normally results in engagement of the frontal plane components of the zygapophyseal joint. An anterior shear stress occurs during weight-bearing at the last two lumbar levels, and these segments are designed to effectively counterbalance this force. Note that an anterior shear force occurs perpendicular to the frontal plane. Only the portion of the inferior articular process that is oriented in the frontal plane engages with the portion of the superior articular process that is also oriented in the frontal plane, and together they minimize the tendency of the fourth lumbar vertebra to slide forward on the fifth lum-

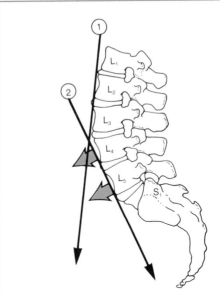

Figure 4–6. Sagittal view of the lumbar spine showing the lumbar lordosis and the difference in the angle of the upper lumbar vertebrae (L1, L2, L3) *(arrow 1)* as compared with the lower two lumbar vertebrae (L4, L5) *(arrow 2)*. This angle change increases the anterior shear force to the L4, L5, and S1 segments.

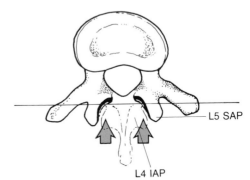

Figure 4–7. Transverse section of the L4-L5 vertebral segment showing a compression or engagement of the frontal plane aspect of the apophyseal joint as the top vertebral body shears anterior.

bar vertebra (Fig. 4–7). The articulation of the fifth lumbar vertebra on the sacrum is stabilized in much the same manner. However, engagement by the joint surfaces is not the only restraint to anterior shear. Table 4–1 lists other

TABLE 4–1.   Structures That Check Anterior Shear of Lumbar Spine

Anterior longitudinal ligament
Anterior height of intervertebral disc at L4 and L5
Annular rings that travel inferior and posterior
Iliolumbar ligament
Frontal plane of apophyseal joint
Muscles that run superior, medial, and anterior (i.e.,
    multifidus, deep iliocostalis, deep longissimus, and
    quadratus lumborum)

structures also oriented to stabilize the lumbar spine against anterior shear. This reiterates the important concept of the synergistic relationship of many tissues in the lumbar spine.

The ligamentum flavum is also the anterior wall of the zygapophyseal joint capsule (Fig. 4–8). It is a highly elastic structure that blends with the extensive fibrous joint capsule. Paris has reviewed these joint capsules in detail.[71] When viewed from the the posterior aspect, the fibers of the capsule run superiorly and medially toward the ligamentum flavum and the interspinous ligament. As with any capsular structure, the direction of the fibers allows movement in some directions more than in others. When combined with the orientation of joint surfaces, the potential for various combinations of motion can be inferred. In the case of the lumbar zygapophyseal joints, the capsular arrangement and joint design are oriented to favor flexion and extension (sagittal plane) motion.

The capsules of the zygapophyseal joints of the lumbar spine are innervated by nerve fibers.[101] Input to the central nervous system from the capsules is presumed to include both nociceptive and proprioceptive afferent nerve fibers by way of the medial branch of the dorsal rami (Chapter 2). As with other synovial joints, the zygapophyseal joints are subject to various pathologies, and the joint capsule and reinforcing connective tissue can be sources of back pain as well as of referred pain into the lower extremity because of the innervation of

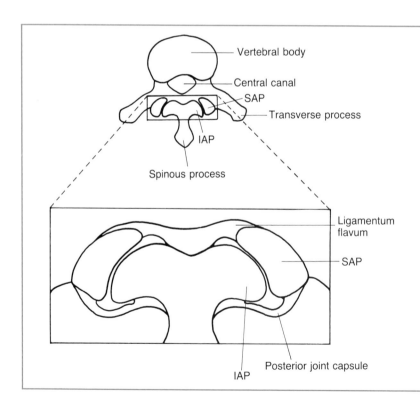

Vertebral body

Central canal
SAP
Transverse process

IAP

Spinous process

Ligamentum
flavum

SAP

Posterior joint capsule

IAP

Figure 4–8. Transverse section of the vertebral segment showing the structure of the apophyseal joint capsule containing the ligamentum flavum anterior and a fibrous capsule posterior.

joint nociceptors.[65] The status of joint position and movement is also relayed from the joints to the central nervous system, triggering reflex motor responses that have yet to be fully elucidated. As mentioned in Chapter 3, the multifidus muscle has attachments to the joint capsule that, theoretically, may provide an additional stimulus to the proprioceptors located in the joint capsule.

ZYGAPOPHYSEAL JOINT MOTION

The plane of the zygapophyseal joints and the orientation of the fibers of the joint capsule and reinforcing ligaments help to dictate the plane of motion for the lumbar spine. As mentioned above, the greatest movement capabili-

ties are in the sagittal plane as compared with the frontal and horizontal planes. The amount of sagittal plane motion has been quantified by numerous investigators demonstrating the large range of movement possible in flexion and extension (Table 4–2). Taylor and Twomey[87,89] note that it is the frontal plane orientation of the articular processes and the fibrous joint capsule that limit anterior shear and forward bending, respectively, during forward bending (Fig. 4–9).

Although sagittal plane motion predominates in the lumbar region, horizontal plane motion is the most limited (Table 4–2). Very simply, the last two lumbar segments are designed to move in the direction of flexion and extension and are not especially designed for rotation. Although some rotation is available, a rotational maneuver, if carried to an extreme,

TABLE 4–2. Representative Values for Range of Motion at Different Segmental Levels of the Spine

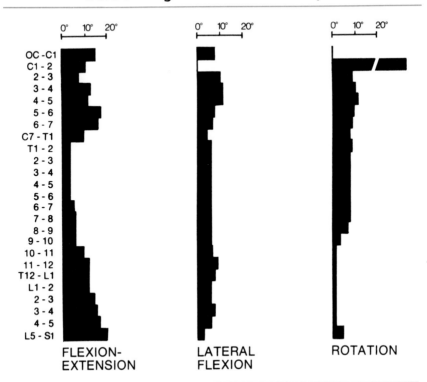

FLEXION-EXTENSION   LATERAL FLEXION   ROTATION

From White and Panjabi: Clinical Biomechanics of the Spine. Philadelphia, J.B. Lippincott Co., 1978.

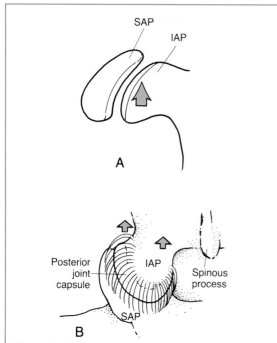

Figure 4–9. *A,* Apophyseal joint surface checks anterior shear. *B,* Posterior view of a left apophyseal joint capsule showing its role in restraining the apophyseal joint in forward bending; IAP moving up on the SAP.

pressive force on the engaged facets, a shear force on the intervertebral disc–vertebral body interface, and a distractive force on the capsular structures on the contralateral side.

The amount of motion in the L4-L5 and L5-S1 regions has been quantified by numerous investigators. Because these lower lumbar segments are the region in which the majority of low back pain occurs, the clinician should be aware of normal movement patterns in this region. There are approximately 20 to 25 degrees of sagittal plane movement between the L4 and L5 vertebrae and the same amount for the L5-S1 segment.[97] This results in these last two segments accounting for nearly 40 to 50 degrees of sagittal plane motion. By comparison, the lower lumbar intervertebral joints have only 3 to 5 degrees of motion in the horizontal plane at each zygapophyseal joint.

Recognizing the limitations of rotation, it would be extremely difficult for the clinician to have a high degree of accuracy in quantifying horizontal plane (rotation) hypomobility, since the total motion is minimal. This is especially true, since it has been estimated that 23 per cent of the apophyseal joints are asymmetrical in the lower lumbar region.[21]

As previously mentioned in the beginning of this chapter, the zygapophyseal joints do not act in isolation from the other structures in the spine. Both the joints and the intervertebral discs contribute to the limitations of segmental motion. However, the intervertebral disc allows movement in many planes owing to the oblique orientation of the collagen fibers of the annular rings (see below), whereas the zygapophyseal joints allow a disproportionate amount of movement in one plane, the sagittal, compared with another, the horizontal.

The analysis of rotation of the lower lumbar joints is interesting from another perspective. Damage to the zygapophyseal joints and the intervertebral disc with excessive torsional forces has been well documented.[3,22] The rotational force places a great deal of compression between the articular cartilage surfaces of the joint. One of the mechanisms the spine has to oppose these torsional forces is the surrounding musculature. The oblique orientation of the muscle fibers of the internal and external abdominal obliques, transversus abdominis,

has the potential to cause damage. During rotation the facet surfaces on one side are placed under compression, whereas on the contralateral side there is a distraction force at the joints.

If an effort is made to continue the rotational movement beyond the available range, an abrupt change in the location of the normal axis of motion for the lumbar spine occurs. Usually the axis of motion for the lumbar spine is in the posterior aspect of the intervertebral disc. However, by engaging the inferior and superior articular processes on one side with the rotational maneuver, the axis shifts further posterior and toward the side of these engaged zygapophyseal joints (Fig. 4–10). With further rotation the vertebral body now pivots around this new axis formed by the engaged joints. This in turn places a shear force on the disc.[7] The extreme rotary motion thus places a com-

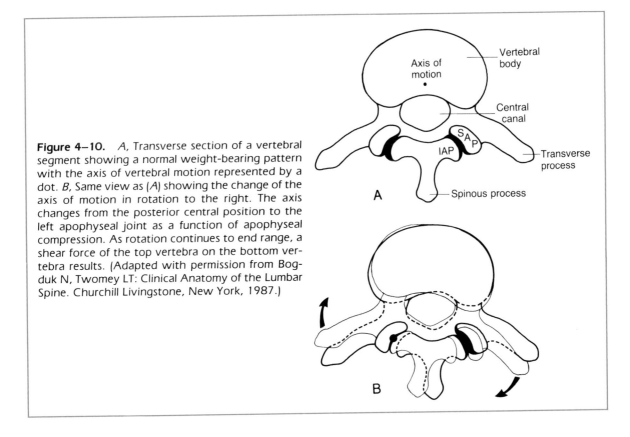

Figure 4–10. *A,* Transverse section of a vertebral segment showing a normal weight-bearing pattern with the axis of vertebral motion represented by a dot. *B,* Same view as (*A*) showing the change of the axis of motion in rotation to the right. The axis changes from the posterior central position to the left apophyseal joint as a function of apophyseal compression. As rotation continues to end range, a shear force of the top vertebra on the bottom vertebra results. (Adapted with permission from Bogduk N, Twomey LT: Clinical Anatomy of the Lumbar Spine. Churchill Livingstone, New York, 1987.)

multifidus, deep erector spinae, quadratus lumborum, and psoas major muscles potentially provides an antitorsion or counterrotation effect in order to counter the torsional force. This stabilizing function might be predicted by analyzing the fiber direction of the various muscles (Fig. 4–11).[74,88] Although there is no scientific evidence to verify that this is one of the muscle's functions, it can be reasonably speculated, if in fact there is synergistic interplay of all the lumbar tissues.

A theoretical stabilizing function becomes even more important when considering the person who attempts to lift an object or move an object overhead. Various combinations of sagittal, frontal, and horizontal plane motions are demanded of the zygapophyseal joints. The weight that is being lifted significantly increases the torque acting at the joints, and there is increased potential for large torque to reach these joints. Adams and Hutton[3] suggest that only a small additional torque to a fully rotated lumbar spine produces damage. The zygapophyseal joint in compression is the first structure to fail at torsional limits, since it is this articulation that offers the primary resistance. The trunk musculature might offer some measure of protection if contraction can be elicited to minimize the torsional forces.

FUNCTIONAL INTERPLAY OF JOINTS AND SURROUNDING TISSUES

Before continuing with the functional aspects of the zygapophyseal joints, the previously introduced concept of an interplay between the joints and the various tissues of the spine should be revisited. Mention has been made of sagittal and horizontal plane motions

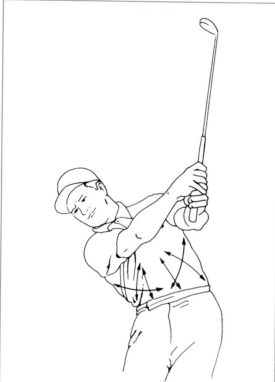

Figure 4–11. Rotational movement of the trunk as in swinging a golf club. The arrows depict the forces generated by the abdominal wall required to stabilize the weight-bearing processes of the spine or counterrotate the trunk.

in order to give the reader the opportunity to visualize joint activity during movement. However, it is important to continually return to this concept of tissue interplay in order to better appreciate the mechanics of movement.

In order to further demonstrate these mechanics, the forward bending motion is briefly discussed. This gives us the opportunity to speculate as to the functional interplay between the zygapophyseal joints, intervertebral disc, and posterior spinal ligaments. Using this example also underscores the fact that lumbar tissues work synergistically during movement patterns to provide for the contradictory demands of mobility and stability.

The example of forward bending is chosen

because of the extent to which this motion is carried out throughout the activities of daily living. As the trunk begins to bend forward from the top down and the motion arrives at the L4 segment, the weight line moves anteriorly, and intradiscal pressure is increased. A compressive force is generated at the anterior aspect of the L4-L5 disc between the L4 and the L5 vertebral bodies. The anterior compressive force generated into this relatively incompressible structure acts now as a fulcrum around which the remainder of the motion can take place (Fig. 4–12).

As the forward motion continues, a tensile stress is imparted to the zygapophyseal joint capsules because of the separation of the articular processes, and the anterior shear stress of the superior vertebrae on the inferior vertebrae increases (see above). This anterior shear is counteracted by the oblique annular rings on

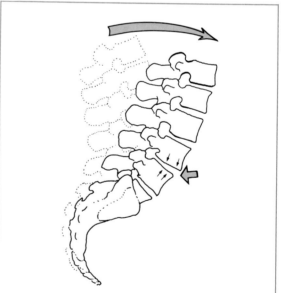

Figure 4–12. Sagittal plane view of the lumbar spine. The dotted lines reveal the starting position, and the solid lines represent a flexed position. Note the arrows portraying a compressive force generated at the anterior disc during flexion. The relatively incompressible intervertebral disc acts as a fulcrum as the motion continues to the next segment.

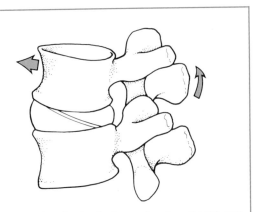

Figure 4–13. Sagittal view of a functional segmental unit showing the inferior and posterior oblique orientation of an annular ring as it checks anterior shear of the top vertebra on the bottom vertebra as flexion continues.

the lateral aspect of the intervertebral disc that travel in a posterior and inferior direction and by the frontal plane orientation of the zygapophyseal joint (Fig. 4–13).[87]

As the fibers of the annular rings become taut, and the articular cartilage of the inferior articulating process of the L4 vertebra engages into the articular cartilage of the superior articulating process of the L5 vertebra, the upward sliding movement at the articular cartilage interface continues. The upward motion of the inferior articulating process is checked by the joint capsule and the posterior ligamentous system.

As the forward bending motion continues, a posterior shear force also occurs in order to provide an equal and opposite counterforce to the anterior shear. This posterior shear force engages the annular fibers that course inferior and anterior, and the interspinous ligament fibers that course superior and posterior. A posterior shear force also occurs owing to the contraction of the deep portion of the iliocostalis lumborum and the lumbar longissimus muscles that are attached to the lumbar transverse processes (see Chapter 3).

These deep erector spinae muscles travel from the iliac crest to the transverse processes of the lumbar vertebrae. They act as lateral guy wires and represent muscle vectors that would be capable of contracting in synchrony to assist in controlling the anterior movement inherent in normal forward bending. This posterior shear exerted actively by contraction of these muscles theoretically decreases the compressive forces exerted by the anterior shear of forward bending on the facet cartilage surfaces that are oriented in the frontal plane. (Fig. 4–14).

As the motion is then transferred down to the next lower segment, the same scenario begins. However, at the L5-S1 segment, the forward shear has another significant check in the form of the iliolumbar ligament.[53] This ligament, with its attachment to the transverse processes of the L5 vertebra, comes into play very quickly to stabilize the segment. As the L5 vertebral body compresses the anterior aspect of the intervertebral disc, the posterior bony elements of the vertebra, which include the transverse processes, are "lifted" upward and anteriorly, away from the iliac crest. This movement results in a tightening of the iliolumbar ligament, thus creating a check to these forces of forward bending.

The mechanics of the L4-L5 segment and the L5-S1 segment are subtly different because of the presence of the iliolumbar ligament at the latter (Fig. 4–15). In the absence of this major passive restraint at the L4-L5 level, there exists the potential for increased anterior shear forces, resulting in increased joint compression (frontal plane). Although this section deals specifically with the example of forward bending, note also that the iliolumbar ligament helps to stabilize the L5-S1 segment in rotation, although this restraint is not afforded the L4-L5 segment. This explanation of the function of these two segments may offer an explanation as to the reason for the increased incidence of injury to the L4-L5 segment.

It should now be better understood how the zygapophyseal joints work in conjunction with many tissues of the lumbar spine during motion. It is also easy to appreciate how altered function of any of these tissues may result in altered mechanics of forward bending (or any other motion) at the zygapophyseal joints.

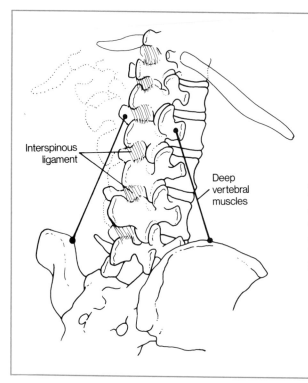

Figure 4–14. Posterior oblique view revealing the role of the posterior vertebral muscles that travel superior, medial, and anterior (two bold lines from ilium to transverse process) and the interspinous ligament, traveling superior and posterior, as they work together with the previously mentioned anatomy to check or counter the anterior shear forces of the lordotic lumbar spine. The vertebrae outlined in dotted lines represent the erect posture, and the vertebrae outlined in bold reveal a slightly flexed posture.

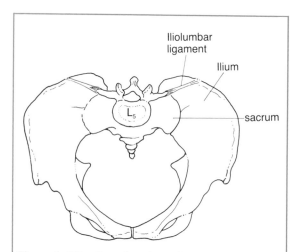

Figure 4–15. Superior view of the L5 vertebra on top of the sacrum and the two paired ilia. Note the lateral extent of the iliolumbar ligament. This is one of the main branches of this ligament. It is designed to stabilize or ''square'' the L5 vertebra on the S1 segment.

WEIGHT-BEARING BY THE ZYGAPOPHYSEAL JOINTS

The zygapophyseal joints have weight-bearing functions, as demonstrated by Adams and Hutton.[2] They note that these joints are responsible for approximately 16 per cent of the weight-bearing load in the upright standing posture, while the remaining load (84 per cent) is borne by the vertebral body–intervertebral disc–vertebral body interface (Fig. 4–16).

This weight-bearing occurs as the inferior articulating process impacts against the superior articulating process. Owing to the normal lumbar lordosis and the frontal plane orientation of the facets of the joint, the anterior aspect of the joint, especially at the last two lumbar levels, experiences a compressive force of weight-bearing. In the standing position the normal lumbar lordosis causes the most anterior aspects of the inferior articulating processes of the lower lumbar segments to impact against the anterior aspect of the superior ar-

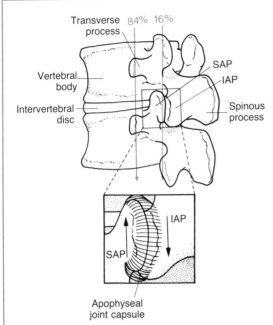

Figure 4–16. *Posterior oblique view of a functional segmental unit with the left apophyseal joint highlighted. Note the arrows that signify 84 per cent weight-bearing properties of the bone-disc-bone interface and the 16 per cent weight-bearing properties of the apophyseal joint. Note in the close-up the posterior aspect of the apophyseal joint capsule as it is utilized in the weight-bearing process.*

ular process glides by the superior articular process. More compressive force occurs between the inferior articular process and the lamina in this case. However, if the superior articular process has a more concave shape, the inferior articular process is compressed into this concave partner.

Like other synovial joints in the body, the zygapophyseal joints have limits in their ability to accept compressive load. The joint surfaces respond with patterns of degeneration as the load exceeds joint limits. For example, rapid impact loading or prolonged, excessive compression has the potential to damage articular cartilage and begin the sequence of joint degeneration.[31,61]

When structural damage to the surface of the articular cartilage occurs, either by injury or by excessive prolonged stress in the upper limits of the physiologic capacity of the joints, the weight-bearing patterns of the joint change.

ticulating processes and the adjacent ligamentum flavum.

As the lumbar spine is extended, weight-bearing by the zygapophyseal joints increases (Fig. 4–17). Instead of sharing the compressive force in the 84 per cent–16 per cent ratio, the proportion of load-sharing between the bone-disc-bone interface and the posterior joints is altered, resulting in an increased compressive force on the joints. As extension increases, the inferior articulating process impacts against the lamina and lower aspect of the superior articular process. If the facet of the superior articular process presents with a flat surface in the portion of the facet oriented in the sagittal plane, minimal weight-bearing occurs between the facets of the joint, since the inferior artic-

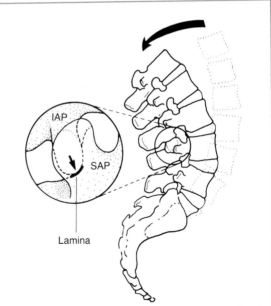

Figure 4–17. *Sagittal view of the lumbar spine in extended posture. Note in close-up the IAP as it impacts against the lamina of the lower aspect of the SAP at the L4-L5 apophyseal joint. This is one of the limiting factors in extension. The dotted line signifies the normal lordotic curve.*

These stresses have the potential to cause further degenerative changes such as denudation of the articular cartilage and eburnation of the subchondral bone.

The weight-bearing limits of the zygapophyseal joint have not been studied in vivo. However, it is worthwhile to consider the potential effect of conditions that may keep the joint excessively loaded. For example, a weak abdominal wall could theoretically alter the way in which forces reach the zygapophyseal joints. This weakness results in an increased anterior tilt of the pelvis, which increases the extension of the lumbar spine (Fig. 4–18). This extension increases the compressive load on the zygapo-

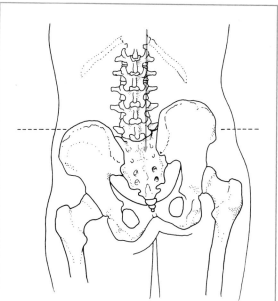

Figure 4–19. A posterior or frontal view of the lumbopelvic region with a left frontal plane asymmetry (sacral tilt down to the left). The arrow signifies the changes of the center of pressure or line of compression as it traverses through the lumbopelvic region. In this example, there is an increased compressive force focused on the right apophyseal joint and right posterior corner of the intervertebral disc. All structures that are designed to stabilize this region become affected by this change in weight-bearing.

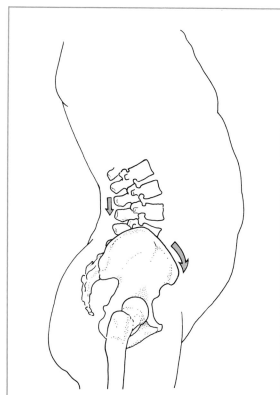

Figure 4–18. Sagittal view of the lumbopelvic region as a result of a weakened abdominal wall. The weakened or lengthened abdominal wall results in an anterior rotary movement on the ilia, which in turn results in extension force at the L4-L5 and L5-S1 apophyseal joints. See arrows.

physeal joints. A relatively shorter leg on one side might also alter the weight-bearing function by positioning the pelvis asymmetrically in the frontal plane. This theoretically places an increased compressive force on the lumbar joints on the side of the relatively longer leg (Fig. 4–19).

Each of these examples is used to enhance the understanding of the weight-bearing function of the zygapophyseal joints. The manner in which the weight line moves through the lumbar spine determines the amount of weight-bearing required by these joints. If ground or trunk forces exceed the physiologic capacity of the joints, degeneration patterns of the hyaline cartilage and subchondral bone of the apophyseal joint may result. Further research is necessary to test these theories.

INTERVERTEBRAL DISC

As previously mentioned, the motion segment for the spine consists of the zygapophyseal joints and the vertebral bodies with the intervertebral disc. Gotfried and associates[29] have stated that the simplistic view that the disc and joints are separate entities is no longer tenable. Forces applied to one must affect the other.

The intervertebral disc can be considered to have two components, the annulus fibrosus and the nucleus pulposus. Because the cartilaginous end plates are intimately related to the intervertebral disc both anatomically and mechanically, they should also be considered during a discussion of the intervertebral disc. Although they do not cover the complete surfaces of the superior and inferior aspects of the intervertebral disc, they are in relation to a significant portion of it. Forces transmitted through the intervertebral disc must have an effect on the cartilaginous end plates. Likewise, forces applied to the cartilaginous end plate reach the intervertebral disc. The first structure to be damaged with excessive compression applied to the vertebral body–intervertebral disc unit is the cartilaginous end plates.[21]

NUCLEUS PULPOSUS

The nucleus pulposus occupies the posterior-central aspect of the intervertebral disc. It consists of mucoid material, cells that resemble chondrocytes, and a loose array of collagen and reticular fibrils. The proteoglycan component of the matrix gives the nucleus pulposus its water-binding capability. As the intervertebral disc ages, the biochemical and histologic makeup of the nucleus changes. There is a decrease in water and proteoglycan components, a change in the types of proteoglycans, and an increase in collagen. Additionally, fibrillation of the nucleus pulposus occurs.

The nucleus pulposus is subjected to cycles of loading and unloading throughout life, which is important for disc nutrition. Degenerative changes that occur in the nucleus are not only caused by the aging process, but also may result from a disturbance in nutrition to the disc. If the loading-unloading cycle is disturbed, the health of the nucleus pulposus can be jeopardized.

Nachemson[66] noted that it is the mechanical loading and unloading of the disc that helps to maintain its health. With only a limited blood supply, especially to the inner aspects of the disc, the continual changeover of fluid in the nucleus—that is, its ability to be hydrated and dehydrated in a cyclical manner—appears important. The health of the nucleus relies on this changeover of fluid, which in turn is facilitated by movement of the spine. The passage of this fluid both into and out of the nucleus pulposus is through the surrounding annulus and especially through the cartilaginous end plates. The importance of the end plates is again noted. They provide an indirect communication link between the rich vascular supply of the cancellous bone of the vertebrae and the central regions of the disc.

ANNULUS FIBROSUS

The annulus fibrosus consists of concentric layers of collagen and fibrous cartilage. If the layers are peeled back from the periphery, it is apparent that the fibers have an oblique orientation. The collagenous fibers in individual lamellae are oriented at approximately a 65-degree angle relative to the axis of the spine (Fig. 4–20).[41] This orients the fibers of the lamellae at approximately 25 degrees with the plateau of the vertebrae. As with any structure that uses collagen, the unit is resistant to tensile stresses. Each layer of the annulus fibrosus is bound to another layer.

The type of collagen in different areas of the annulus is also region-specific. Brickley-Parsons and Glimcher[11] have shown that type 1 and type 2 collagen occupy specific regions of the intervertebral disc. There is a remodeling process that occurs from adolescence to early

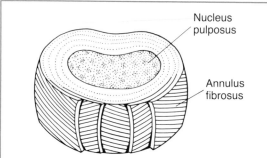

Figure 4–20. Anterosuperior view of the intervertebral disc showing a cross section of the anterior lamina. This view reveals a 65-degree angle relation from one annular ring to the other.

adulthood that results in a different collagenous makeup on the posterior aspect of the lumbar discs (compression region) as compared with the anterior aspect of the disc (tensile region). This remodeling process is a type of redistribution of collagen based on imposed demand.

The oblique orientation of the collagen fibers changes during spinal motion. As the disc becomes compressed, for example, the orientation of the fibers is altered so that the fibers become more horizontal (Fig. 4–21). This means that the collagen fibers become closer to parallel with the vertebral body as axial compression forces are placed on the disc.[48]

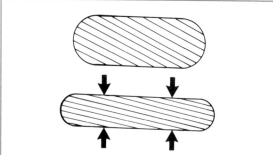

Figure 4–21. Side view of an annular ring as it becomes compressed. The direction of the annular fibers becomes more horizontal as the compressive forces enter the annular ring.

Likewise, bending and torsional movements cause a reorientation of the collagen fibers (Fig. 4–22).[49] In forward bending the posterior annulus is stretched, the anterior annulus is slackened, and the collagen fibers coursing anteriorly and superiorly on the lateral aspect of the disc are subject to increased tension. In a like manner, torsion causes a strain on the collagen fibers that are oriented in one particular direction, but slackens the fibers that are oriented in an opposite direction.

In addition, the annulus is thicker in the anterior and lateral regions and thinner posteriorly. This may be due to the eccentric position of the nucleus, which requires the posterior layers to occupy less surface area than the anterior or lateral layers. Markolf and Morris[57] state that the posterior annular rings have less binding substances between them. The posterior aspect of the annular rings are thinner and not as firmly held together, which may make them more vulnerable to degeneration.

CARTILAGINOUS END PLATES

Because the intervertebral disc is predominantly an avascular structure, it is largely dependent on the passive diffusion of nutrients through the cartilaginous end plates. In addition to this contribution, however, the cartilaginous end plate provides a barrier that minimizes the possibility for loss of proteoglycans from the intervertebral disc.[10]

Besides contributing to this nutritive function, the cartilaginous end plates are involved with the mechanics of the spine. They provide a physical barrier for the nucleus pulposus into the vertebral body, and the end plate also distributes part of the hydrostatic pressure exerted on it by the nucleus pulposus. The collagen fibers of the end plate are oriented horizontally; this allows conjecture as to how this design is optimal for resisting the forces that would be exerted against it by the pressure of the nucleus (Fig. 4–23). Bulging of the nucleus would have a "bowing" effect on the cartilaginous end plate. This "bowing" produces a tensile force on the end plate, in much the same manner as the tensile forces are im-

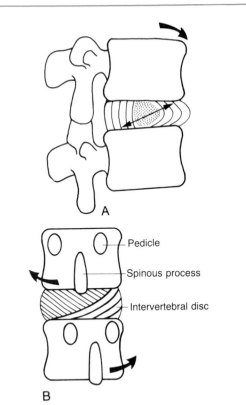

Figure 4-22. *A,* Sagittal view of the functional segmental unit depicting the forces and stresses on the intervertebral disc in forward bending. The collagenous structures of the annulus fibrosus of the intervertebral disc adapt to this position by an increased tensile force to the posterior aspect of the disc and increased compressive force anteriorly. The arrow within the intervertebral disc signifies the annular ring that travels inferior and posterior as it checks anterior shear, a resultant force of forward bending. *B,* Posterior view of a functional segmental unit showing the reorientation of the collagenous fibers of the annulus in rotation to the right. Note the tightening of the fibers traveling in one direction and the loosening of the fibers traveling in the opposite direction. It should be recognized that rotation also includes compression.

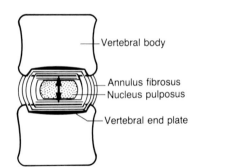

Figure 4-23. Bone-disc-bone interface showing the relation of the annular rings and nucleus pulposus as they interrelate with the vertebral end plates. Note how this design is optimal for resisting forces that would be exerted against it by the nucleus pulposus.

continuous with the intervertebral disc. The collagen fibers of the disc continue into the end plate by turning approximately 120 degrees from the lamellae of the outer annulus and 90 degrees from the nucleus.[78] The chemical components of the end plate are also similar to those of the intervertebral disc: proteoglycans, collagen, and water. These three key chemical components are present in the end plate, annulus fibrosus, and nucleus pulposus, but in different proportions. The different proportions ultimately contribute to the physical and functional differences of the intervertebral disc and the cartilaginous end plate.

INTERVERTEBRAL DISC MECHANICS

The nucleus normally remains confined within the surrounding annulus fibrosus and the superior and inferior cartilaginous end plates. There is no clear demarcation between the inner annulus fibrosus and the outer nucleus pulposus. It is, therefore, unreasonable to think of the nucleus pulposus as a completely distinct spherical unit in the center of the annulus. Because the two structures blend together, it is impossible for the nucleus pulposus to "move" en masse in any direction.

parted to young bone in greenstick fractures. By orienting the collagen fibers horizontally, the tensile forces are resisted, and the end plate supports the hydrostatic pressure.[78]

Anatomically, the cartilaginous end plate is

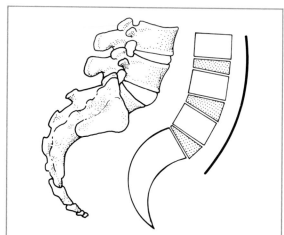

Figure 4–24. Sagittal view of the L4-L5 and sacral segments on the left and an artist's rendition on the right. Note that at the L4-L5 and L5-S1 segments the intervertebral disc is wedge-shaped and often twice the height anteriorly as posteriorly.

The intervertebral discs between L4-L5 and between L5-S1 are wedge-shaped. The anterior height of the L5-S1 disc is often twice the height of the posterior aspect (Fig. 4–24). This shape is one of the major reasons for the existence of lumbar lordosis.[21] The disc between the L3-L4 vertebrae has a more evenly distributed anterior and posterior height relation.

Considering the shape of these two discs and recognizing the mechanical properties of collagen, it is apparent that it is difficult to compress the anterior height to such an extent that the posterior height becomes much greater than the anterior height. Pearcy and Tibrewal[72] have shown this with standing full flexion and full extension radiographs.

Some mechanical models of the disc that argue for the nucleus moving in a backward direction show a disc with equal anterior and posterior heights. Furthermore, these mechanical models assume that when the spine is flexed, collapse of the anterior aspect causes a force that pushes the nucleus posteriorly. Because the lower two lumbar discs are more wedge-shaped, this is clearly not the mechanical behavior of the lower lumbar intervertebral discs, where in fact most disc lesions occur. The anterior height remains greater

than or equal to the posterior height in full flexion, and consequently a unidirectional, posteriorly directed force on the nucleus owing to collapse of the anterior aspect of the disc does not develop. However, alteration in intradiscal pressure with spine motion does occur, which is the more critical issue.

Nachemson and Morris[67] measured the pressure developed in the disc under various compressive forces, and because the needle was inserted into the nucleus pulposus region, intradiscal pressure has come to be synonymous with the pressure within the nucleus pulposus. These experiments shed great light on force transmission through the intervertebral disc. They demonstrated that forces were transferred into the disc as body positions were changed.

Rather than thinking of the nucleus as a mass pushing in one particular direction, the nucleus should be viewed as a structure that is exerting forces in all directions (Fig. 4–25). This is logical, since the nucleus imbibes water and, as a result, develops an internal pressure. The pressure exerted is in all directions, and includes lateral forces exerted against the an-

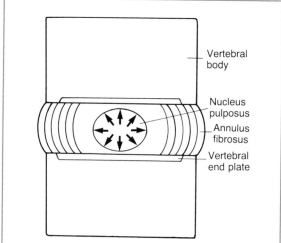

Figure 4–25. Bone-disc-bone interface showing the annulus, vertebral end plates, and nucleus of the intervertebral disc. Note that the nucleus exerts pressure in all directions as forces are exerted into and through it.

nulus and superiorly and inferiorly directed forces against the cartilaginous end plates. It is as if every point on a sphere is exerting an exploding force. This force is essentially equal in all directions.

Note, however, that different body positions can influence the total compressive force being exerted on the intervertebral disc. Besides the changes in body position themselves, intradiscal pressure also increases as a result of the contraction of the muscles surrounding the spine. Total intradiscal pressure is a summation of the pressures generated as a result of spine positioning and muscle contraction.

This is different than saying that the nucleus pulposus is the component of the intervertebral disc that absorbs compressive forces. The annulus fibrosus is actually the structure more adept at accepting compressive forces. Markolf and Morris[57] and Virgin[90] demonstrated that enucleated discs respond very nearly the same as discs with the nucleus pulposus intact when compressive forces were applied for a short period. This means that disc deformation curves caused by increasing compression stresses are essentially the same whether the nucleus pulposus is present or not.

Compression of the disc does not cause extrusion of the normal nucleus even in experiments in which the annulus is intentionally damaged and compression forces are applied.[90] Instead, it is the cartilaginous end plates that rupture. In order for the nucleus pulposus to escape the confines of the annulus fibrosus, two conditions must exist:

1. The wall of the annulus must weaken. This can be due to injury that decreases the stiffness of the annular rings. The posterior aspect of the annulus is particularly susceptible to this, since it has less mass.

2. The proteoglycan content of the nucleus pulposus is no longer able to hold the nuclear matrix together, and the nucleus pulposus becomes partially desiccated. This may occur with mechanical stresses, but it is most likely to occur as a result of biochemical changes within the nucleus itself. Strong evidence exists for the protein of the nucleus pulposus to serve as an antigenic agent.[58] An autoimmune reaction, with its attendant inflammatory re-

sponse, may contribute to breakdown of the nucleus pulposus. This antibody–antigen reaction perhaps occurs as a result of defects in the cartilaginous end plate from various mechanical insults. With the barrier between the nucleus pulposus and the rich circulation of the vertebral body disrupted, the protein of the nucleus pulposus is exposed to the circulating antibodies and may, theoretically, trigger such a response.

The pathology of intervertebral disc injury is discussed below. However, it is addressed at this point in order to provide detail regarding intervertebral disc mechanics.

Let us return to the concept of intradiscal pressure. This pressure exerts superiorly and inferiorly directed forces that essentially attempt to push the vertebrae "apart," and horizontally directed forces that push against the annulus. The effect of these forces is to increase the stiffness of the cartilaginous end plate and the annulus fibrosus.

Why is the nucleus pulposus exerting this outward pressure? We speculate as to some possible reasons.

By exerting this positive pressure, the nucleus pulposus is actually pushing the vertebrae apart. This may have several effects. First, the zygapophyseal joints are potentially unloaded, or more accurately, they are subject to less compressive force (Fig. 4–26). Although they are weight-bearing structures, they are responsible for only a small proportion of weight-bearing. Dunlop and coworkers[18] have shown experimentally that peak pressure between the zygapophyseal joints increases significantly with loss of disc height and with increasing extension. These higher contact pressures could possibly damage the facet articular surfaces and result in degenerative disease of the lumbar joints.

Therefore, this first role of the nucleus may be mechanical in nature, that is, to help unload the zygapophyseal joints. Gotfried and colleagues[29] have suggested a cause-and-effect relation between disc space narrowing and zygapophyseal joint degeneration.

A second role may be neurologic in nature. By having a structure that causes a distraction force to the vertebral elements, a certain tension develops within the supporting connec-

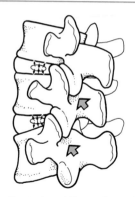

Figure 4–26. Posterior oblique view of the L3, L4, and L5 segments showing the positive pressure of the nucleus pulposus that not only unloads the zygapophyseal joint (see arrows), but also maintains the size and shape of the neuroforamen.

alized afferent input into the central nervous system. Our proposal is that the nucleus pulposus contributes to this afferent neurologic input by affecting tension in the surrounding connective tissues, thus influencing the mechanoreceptor system.

The third role relates to increasing the ring stiffness of the annulus fibrosus. The nucleus pulposus exerts pressure against the walls of the annulus fibrosus. By having this pressure exerted, a tensile force on the annular rings results (Fig. 4–27). This tensile force results in an increased stiffness of the annulus. The increased stiffness in turn makes the annulus better able to absorb compression stresses that are applied for extended time periods, helping to avoid collapse of the annulus. The increased stiffness also allows the annulus to more effectively restrict and regulate movement of the vertebrae.

tive tissue structures. Wyke[100] has shown the capsular tissue to be rich with various types of mechanoreceptors and nociceptors, while Malinksy[56] has demonstrated the presence of nerve fibers in the outer aspect of the annulus fibrosus. Gracovetsky and Farfan[30] have suggested that these receptors may be more completely viewed as stress receptors, since they are biologic transducers recording the various stresses placed on these connective tissue structures.

The distraction force exerted by the nucleus pulposus helps to place these tissues at a certain preset tension. This tension stimulates the stress receptors, which in turn starts a centripetal flow of afferent information to the central nervous system. By the nucleus pulposus exerting this pressure and helping to maintain this slight preset tension on the surrounding tissues, small movements in any of these innervated tissues further stimulate the receptors because of their distortion. This increases the barrage of signals into the central nervous system, which in turn can result in a variety of reflex motor responses.

The wide range of postures and movement patterns used in lifting, for example, points out that each person's efferent motor output is subject to variations. These variations in turn are probably caused by the unique and individu-

PATHOLOGY OF INTERVERTEBRAL DISC INJURY

The annulus fibrosus must withstand the multiple stresses that arise from compression, torsion, bending, and shear. From a structural standpoint, it appears that the posterior aspect of the annulus is most vulnerable to damage.[12] The posterior region is narrower and the lamellae are thinner. Consequently damage can readily occur in this region.

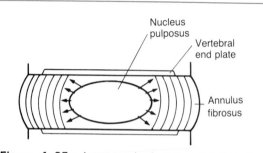

Figure 4–27. Intervertebral disc, depicting the third role related to the positive pressure of the nucleus pulposus (i.e., increasing the ring stiffness of the annulus fibrosus).

Annular injury is the important first step in initiating disc pathology. Once the annular rings are "softened," overstretched, or torn owing to the normal viscoelasticity being exceeded, they are no longer as effective in stabilizing or limiting the motion of the vertebral bodies and in containing the pressure of the nucleus. The pressure by the nucleus pulposus is now exerted against an area of less resistance. As a result, buckling of the annulus occurs, resulting in the well-known disc bulge.

If the nucleus pulposus becomes fragmented, the nuclear material can "dissect" its way through breaches in the annulus fibrosus, resulting in extrusion. There is a gradual leaking of desiccated nuclear material toward the defect in the annulus. Interestingly, Hampton and associates[37] have shown that an annular defect in the shape of a fissure has limited healing potential and can provide a pathway for irritating nuclear fluid to escape onto perineural tissue, possibly resulting in persistent and chronic low back pain. This is in direct contrast to experimentally induced "pluglike" deficits, which heal with a solid block of fibrous tissue.

If we now combine postural positions (that have a high intradiscal pressure) with spine motion, then movement of nuclear material is enhanced because it is under high pressure. The younger, gel-like nucleus pulposus is more effective in exerting a higher pressure against the annular walls when compared with the older nucleus, which is more fibrous and has more collagen. These age-related changes of the nucleus pulposus help to explain why disc pathology is more common in young adults (20 to 40 years old) than in the elderly.

However, disc protrusions (bulge at the level of the intervertebral disc), prolapses (contents of the disc have escaped into the epidural space but there is still continuity with the involved disc), or extrusions (extruded material has lost continuity with the involved disc) are not limited to nucleus pulposus tissue. Yasuma and coworkers[102] have noted that the herniated disc material can be composed of nucleus pulposus, annulus fibrosus, or a combination of the two. A close look at their data shows that cartilaginous end plate material also contributes to some of the herniations.

What types of force cause this breach or weakening of the annulus that precipitates nuclear herniation? There are many potential insults. The annular lesion may be the result of a lifetime of abnormal stresses to the annulus. It may also weaken because of isolated trauma, such as excessive torsion to the spine, prolonged periods of vibration, and excessive and prolonged loading. Etiologic factors such as these result in the viscoelasticity of the annular collagen being exceeded.

Prolonged extension stresses—for example, in excessive lordotic posturing—might place greater than normal compressive forces on the inherently weaker posterior annulus. This in turn may result in structural fatigue of the collagen, and ultimately may weaken the fibers, making them more susceptible to injury.

Torsional forces can damage the collagen fibers of the annulus. Torsion applied to the disc would submit the oblique collagen fibers to forces that would tend to increase their length. When these torsional forces are applied, half of the fibers go through this elongation motion, since successive annular layers are oriented perpendicular to overlying and underlying layers. Stated another way, a torsional force will cause a tensile stress on half of the fibers and relaxation of the remaining fibers. From this point the analogy with any ligamentous tissue in the body can be made. If the viscoelasticity of the fiber under tensile stress is exceeded, permanent elongation or collagen fiber tearing occurs. The stiffness, normally imparted by the connective tissue of annulus, is now lessened by the injury.

Fatigue loading of the collagen of the annulus might also occur as a result of excessive forward bending forces, which places tensile stresses on the posterior annular wall. Repeated forward bending might result in structural fatigue of the collagen located in the posterior aspect of the annulus fibrosus. A sudden, high-velocity force that exceeds the elastic component of the collagen might also damage the posterior aspect of the annulus. In either case, the lamellae of the annulus are sufficiently distorted to render it structurally weaker.[59]

The annular injury that might occur as a result of forward bending, or forward bending with combined torsion of the trunk, is difficult to distinguish clinically from other soft-tissue sprains and strains. During a forward bending motion the axis of rotation is in the region of the nucleus. As the motion proceeds, the instantaneous center of rotation gradually moves anteriorly. Regardless of the exact position of this axis, all structures that are posterior to the axis of rotation must elongate. Those tissues furthest from the axis must go through a greater lengthening than the tissues closest to the axis (Fig. 4–28).

As a result, any tissue posterior to the axis might be injured. This would include all tissues from the posterior annular fibers at the central core of the spine out to the skin and fascia at the most superficial aspect of the posterior trunk. Clinically, many of these tissues, including the annulus, joint capsules, muscles, and fascia, have the capability to give rise to

referred pain if they are injured. Therefore, distinguishing the annular lesion from injury to any other tissue is oftentimes difficult.

Positioning the patient who has incurred this forward bending injury in a posture that extends the lumbar spine has the effect of removing the tensile forces on all structures posterior to the axis of rotation. This is an effective way to rest or immobilize tissue. As a result, the referral pain pattern may diminish because injured tissue is not held in an elongated position. To attribute pain relief only to altered disc mechanics ignores all of the other tissues of the spine.

Increases in muscle strength or increases in hip or low back flexibility do not alter the actual pathology of the disc lesion. However, they may affect the pathogenesis of disc lesions. To do so, the changes in strength or length must alter the way in which forces reach the disc. Whether the person is standing, sitting, or moving, the weight line must be controlled. Controlling the weight line means the transference of forces through the lumbopelvic region in a nondestructive manner. It is important that the forces reaching the intervertebral disc are not excessive in order to avoid damage.

Likewise, movement patterns such as those used in lifting, carrying, or reaching must occur in such a manner that abnormal forces do not reach the annulus. In the discussion of the zygapophyseal joints an antitorsion role was predicted for various trunk musculature owing to their oblique orientation. The same function can be recognized relative to the disc. These muscles are oriented to help prevent excessive torsional movements from reaching the intervertebral disc.

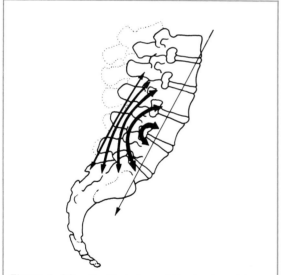

Figure 4–28. Sagittal view of the lumbopelvic region. The dotted lines represent the starting position, and the solid lines of the vertebral segments indicate a forward bend position. The arrows that proceed from the center of rotation posteriorward indicate the extent the tissues must go through as the lumbar spine foward bends. The tissues farthest from the axis of rotation (posterior aspect of the intervertebral disc) experience the greatest excursion.

THE SACROILIAC JOINTS

The two paired sacroiliac joints have been the source of considerable controversy for many decades as well as the subject of many studies. The reader is referred to studies published more than 50 years ago in order to gain an appreciation of the historical perspective.[1,13,73,79] The sacroiliac joint has long been used by anthropologists as a skeletal target to determine the age of the specimen. It is well accepted that the joint is an extremely stable structure because of its bony configuration and ligamentous support. There are recorded cases in which severe trauma caused fractures of the ilium and sacrum, but failed to disrupt the sacroiliac joints.[14] The ligaments of this joint are among the strongest in the human body.[99]

Considerable effort has been expended to quantify the normal range of movement of the sacroiliac joint and to apply this information to treatment approaches.[14,17,19,25,34,51,54,55,63,64,80,84,85,94,95] Mitchell[64] suggests that the ilium rotates in a posterior direction at heel strike and progressively moves in an anterior direction as the person passes through stance phase. He describes the movement of the sacrum on the ilium as occurring around three horizontal axes, a view different from that of Weisl,[94] who identified oblique axes around which the sacrum and ilium move. Colachis and coworkers[14] used pins placed in the pelvic bones to determine movement. Their conclusions noted that there is a small amount of movement present, with the greatest amount occurring in the position of forward bending from the standing position. Weisl[94] reported movement of 5.6 mm, whereas Sashin[79] reported an average range of 4 degrees of movement between the sacrum and ilium. Sturesson and associates[85] found even less movement with a sophisticated roentgen stereophotogrammetric analysis. That the movements are small is fairly well accepted. The controversial aspect is related to the significance of this small amount of potential motion.

The sacrum is influenced by movements that direct forces to it from above through the lumbar spine. These forces have been described in Chapter 1 as trunk forces (Fig. 4–29). The innominate bones are also governed by forces that reach them by way of the lower extremities and act through the hip joint. These have been referred to in Chapter 1 as ground forces (Fig. 4–30).

When these forces reach the pelvis (for the purpose of clarity, pelvis refers to the innominate bones and sacrum), they must be attenuated by the joints and supporting tissues. The

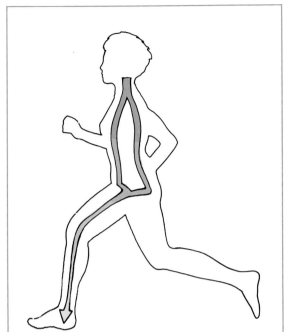

Figure 4–29. *Trunk forces.* Attenuation of trunk forces as they begin at the head and travel inferior toward the ground. The shaded area shows the force attenuation functions of our musculoskeletal system (i.e., as the force travels toward the ground, it becomes less).

applied stresses must also be within the limits of physiologic tolerances. However, when these stresses exceed the normal physiologic capacity of the tissues, an injury with a resultant painful condition can develop.[6,15,20,28] The exact mechanism of lesions to this region has been quite controversial. In order to better formulate thoughts as to possible mechanisms of injury, the anatomy of the sacroiliac joint should be detailed.

Anatomy

The innominate bone is composed of three segments: the ilium, ischium, and pubis. The paired innominates provide four surface projections that can serve as landmarks for palpation.[40] These landmarks are the anterior su-

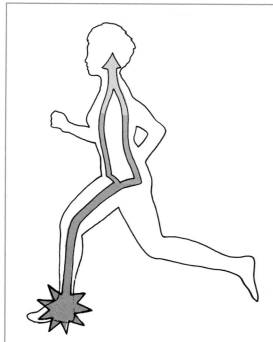

Figure 4–30. *Ground forces.* Impact or ground reaction forces as they travel through the lower extremity and into and through the trunk. (Adapted with permission from Porterfield JP, DeRosa C: The Sacroiliac Joint in Orthopaedic and Sports Physical Therapy, second edition, ed. Gould JA, C.V. Mosby, St. Louis, 1990.)

perior iliac spine, the iliac crest, the posterior superior iliac spine, and the pubic tubercle (Fig. 4–31). The ilium is the portion of the innominate that articulates with the sacrum to form the sacroiliac joint, and thus the terms iliosacral and sacroiliac are appropriate anatomical terms for this joint.

The sacrum is a mass of irregularly shaped bone formed by the fusion of five sacral vertebrae and perforated by four pairs of neuroforamina. Solonen[82] has found that approximately 87 per cent of the articular surface of the sacroiliac joint is formed by the first, second, and third sacral segments. The sacrum is wider superiorly than inferiorly, and broader anteriorly than posteriorly (Fig. 4–32). Its overall shape roughly resembles a truncated pyramid with the base located superiorly and anteriorly.

The body of the S1 vertebra articulates with the body of the L5 vertebra by way of the lumbar intervertebral disc, facilitating the transmission of weight from the trunk to the pelvis. Posteriorly, the zygapophyseal joints link the two segments. The plane of the zygapophyseal joints between L5 and S1 varies from person to person and can also be asymmetrical when comparing the right side to the left. The orientation is usually a combination of the frontal and sagittal planes.[87]

The two sacroiliac joints are L- or auricular-

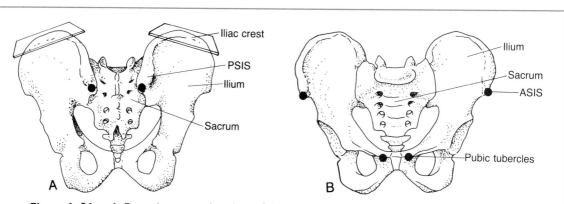

Figure 4–31. *A,* Frontal or posterior view of the pelvis outlining two palpation points, the iliac crest (plane) and the posterior superior iliac spines (PSIS) (black dots). *B,* Anterior view of the pelvis showing bony landmarks, the anterior superior iliac spines (ASIS) (superior black dots) and the pubic tubercles (inferior black dots). These points are readily palpated during the examination process.

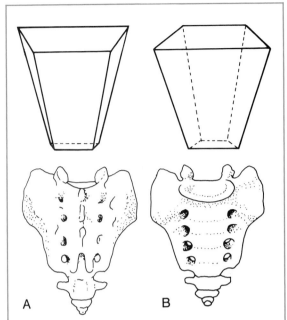

Figure 4–32. *A*, Posterior view of the sacrum and drawing of a truncated pyramid showing the sacrum to be wider superiorly than inferiorly. *B*, Anterior view of the sacrum (inferior) and drawing of a truncated pyramid (superior) indicating that the sacrum is wider anteriorly than posteriorly.

shaped when viewed from the side (Fig. 4–33). Their surfaces are divided into cranial and caudal segments, with the caudal usually being larger.[5,9,94] Weisl's[94] extensive studies of these joints have shown that a central tubercle can often be found at the junction of the cranial and caudal segments on the sacrum, which fits into a central depression in the same location on the ilium.

The sacral component of the joint is concave and lined with hyaline cartilage that is 1.7 to 5 times thicker than the fibrocartilage that covers the convex iliac component.[6,9] The iliac component is usually convex and lined with a thin fibrocartilage. As these two joint partners articulate and become compressed, cartilage deformation results. This accommodation by the cartilage is one method of force attenuation by the sacroiliac joint as trunk and ground forces converge into the region.

Figure 4–34 reveals a transverse section of the sacrum at three cross-sectional levels. The reader should note the differences in the topography and the space between the cartilaginous surfaces at each level of the sacral and iliac components. The configuration and location of the extensive interosseous ligament should also be noted. This thick fibrous ligament, attached to both bones, fills a large portion of the cavity that is formed as the ilium meets the sacrum. The ligament provides stability to the sacroiliac joint and at the same time permits small, deforming, translational movements of the ilium and sacrum on each other as trunk and ground forces converge into the region.

The contour of the sacroiliac joint changes as we go through the aging process.[6,9,70,79,93] The joint surfaces remain flat until sometime after puberty. During the third and fourth decades there is an increase in the size and number of elevations and depressions on the sacral and iliac surfaces, which forms an interlocking system and limits mobility between the two bones. The curves and irregularities are greater in the male, and the formation of fibrous adhesions with gradual obliteration of a true joint space occurs in both sexes. This obliteration occurs earlier in males and after menopause in females.[99] There is a decrease in mobility owing to the initial stages of joint fibrosis that become evident in the third and fourth decades.[5,9,79]

Besides the bony architecture, stability of the pelvis is also due to strong supporting ligaments. The sacroiliac joint is reinforced by the anterior and posterior sacroiliac ligaments and the previously mentioned interosseous ligament. The posterior sacroiliac ligaments are extremely thick and stronger than the anterior sacroiliac ligaments.

The sacrotuberous and sacrospinous ligaments are attached to the sacrum and ischium. Their function becomes evident in weight-bearing positions because they act to check the forward flexion moment of the sacrum on the innominate as trunk forces converge on the sacrum. They also minimize the potential for one ilium to rotate posteriorly on the sacrum owing to the orientation of the ligament. These ligaments are further discussed below.

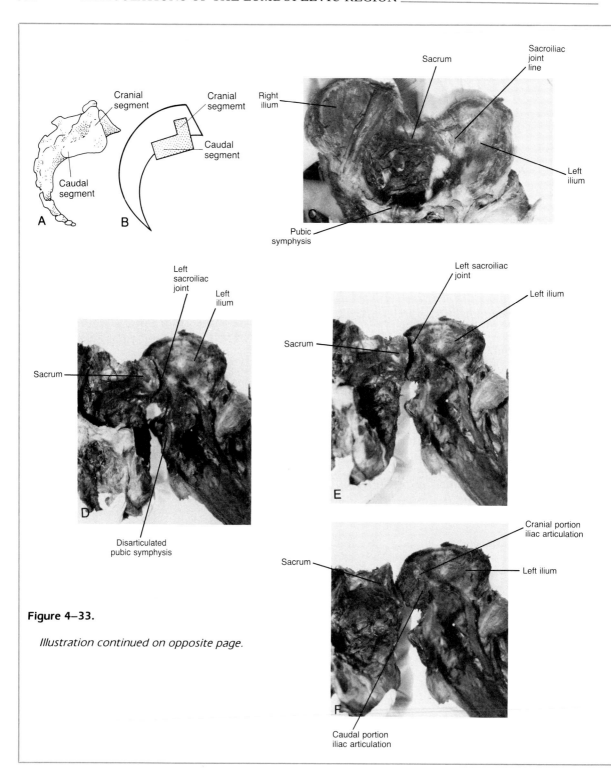

Figure 4–33.

Illustration continued on opposite page.

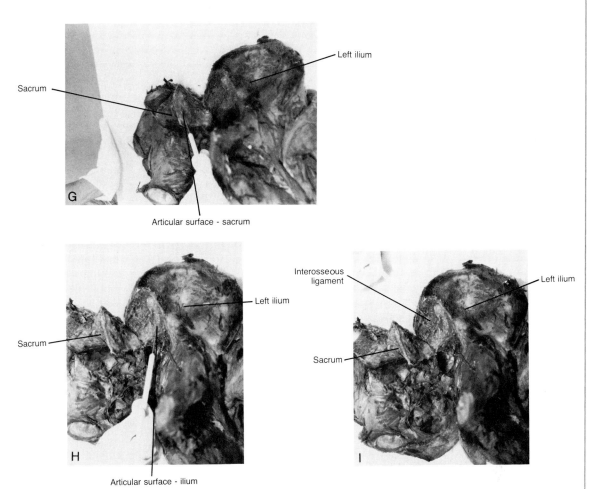

Figure 4–33. *A*, Sagittal view of the sacrum showing the sacroiliac articulation. *B*, Sacroiliac surface showing the cranial and caudal segments of the sacroiliac articulation as an L-shaped surface. *C*, Superior view of a cadaver section showing the sacrum, the pubic symphysis, and the two paired ilia. The lumbar spine has been removed. *D*, More anterior view of the same section with a disarticulated pubic symphysis showing a slight disarticulation of the left sacroiliac joint. *E*, Continued lateral disarticulation of the left sacroiliac joint with an enlarged view of the articular surface. The ilial portion is mainly seen in this view. *F*, Completely disarticulated left sacroiliac joint. The ilial and sacral components can be seen. Note the L shape and the cranial and caudal portions of the ilial surface. *G*, Close-up view of the disarticulated left sacroiliac joint. The probe is placed on the sacral component of the sacroiliac joint. The hyaline cartilage lining this joint is three to five times thicker than the fibrocartilaginous surface of the ilial component. Note the irregular topography of this joint. *H*, Left disarticulated sacroiliac joint with the probe placed at the apex of the cranial and caudal segments of the ilial portion of the sacroiliac joint. *I*, Left disarticulated joint with the probe placed at the posterior aspect of the ilial surface, indicating the position of the interosseous ligament. This ligament is placed between the ilium and the sacrum posterior to the joint surface.

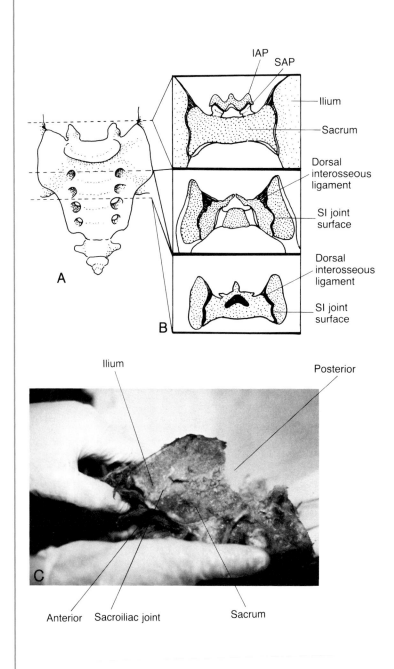

Figure 4–34. *A,* Anterior view of the sacrum and partial drawing of the ilia bilateral. The dotted lines signify transverse sections to be seen in *B. B,* Transverse section of the first sacral segment—note the L5-S1 apophyseal joint; the second sacral segment—note the depth of the dorsal interosseous ligament and joint surfaces, convex/concave; and the third sacral segment—note the interosseous ligament and the sacroiliac joint surface. *C,* A transverse section of a cadaver specimen through the second sacral segment. Note the anterior and posterior orientation, and the ilium on the left and the sacrum on the right in the sacroiliac joint surface. *D,* A transverse section of the cadaver segment at the second sacral level. The probe is indicating the interosseous ligament. From an anterior to posterior relationship, the tissues that lie on top of this ligament are the posterior sacroiliac ligaments, the multifidus muscle, the aponeurosis of the superficial erector spinae, the posterior layer of the thoracolumbar fascia, the subcutaneous fat, and then the skin. *E,* A transverse section of the cadaver segment at the second sacral level. The probe is indicating the sacroiliac joint surface. Notice the convex/concave relationship as well as the thicker hyaline cartilage on the sacral surface. *F,* A transverse section of a cadaver specimen at the second sacral segment revealing a disarticulated sacroiliac joint. Note the hand-in-glove relationship of the two joint surfaces as well as the significance of the interosseous ligament with respect to stability of this region.

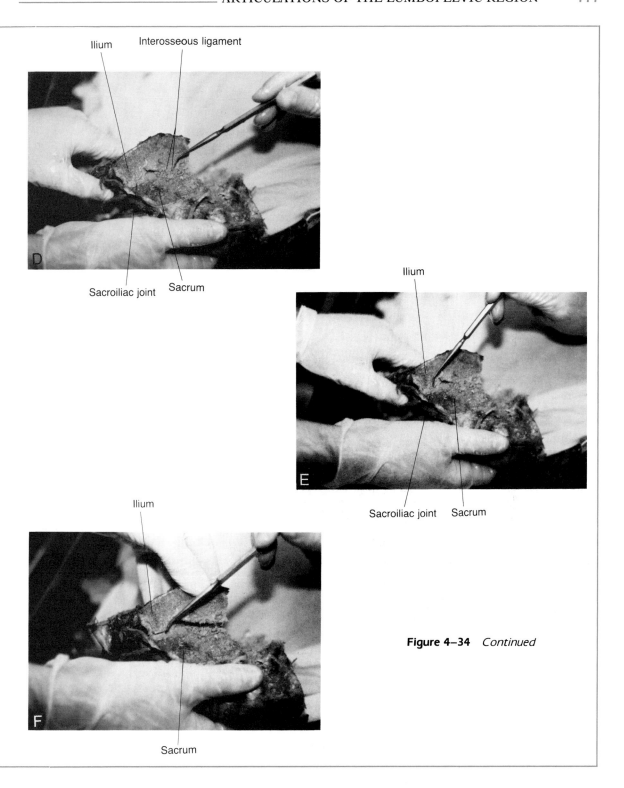

Figure 4–34 *Continued*

Biomechanics

The biomechanics of the female pelvis are different than those of the male pelvis. Structurally, the female pelvis is shorter and wider than the male pelvis. The hormonal changes of menses and pregnancy render the female pelvis slightly more mobile, and it has been suggested that this results in an increased vulnerability to soft-tissue injury.[8,23,28] Initially Hishaw[39] and later Weiss[96] described the release of the hormone relaxin during pregnancy. The titer of this hormone, probably in combination with other biochemical changes, appears to alter the stiffness of the connective tissue so that increased motion is available to allow for expansion of the pelvic outlet and to facilitate the passage of the infant through the birth canal. The ischial tuberosities are initially closer together before the infant has moved into the pelvic canal. However, as the infant moves down the pelvic canal, the ischial tuberosities spread, causing an inward motion of the ilia.

Although the biochemical changes may facilitate childbirth, they may potentially render the weight-bearing joints of the pelvis vulnerable to sprain because of excessive motion. This may also include the period during which the infant is breastfed, which also features biochemical changes. Specific sacroiliac joint injury related to pregnancy, therefore, can occur before, during, or for a time after childbirth.

The subject of movement of the sacroiliac joint remains controversial.[17,19,47,51,85] The concept of normal physiologic movement of the female pelvis during parturition is well accepted, but the physiologic movements of the male and female sacroiliac joints during functional activities have led to lively debate in the literature.

Because of the attachments of the sacrum within the pelvis and to the fifth lumbar vertebra, forward motion (reducing the lumbar lordosis) and backward motion (increasing the lumbar lordosis) result in forces on the sacrum. For example, while bending the lumbar spine (specifically L5) forward at the lumbosacral junction, there must be a counterbalancing force at the sacrum. This counterbalance is mainly provided by the contraction of the glu-

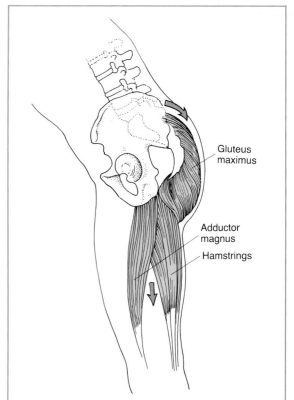

Figure 4–35. Sagittal view of the lumbopelvic region showing the force generated by the contraction of the gluteus maximus, hamstrings, and posterior portion of the adductor magnus, causing a posterior rotary force of the pelvis that counterbalances the forces of forward bending.

teus maximus, hamstrings, and posterior portion of the adductor magnus muscles as they pull downward on the pelvis (with its component sacrum), causing a posterior rotation of the pelvis around the hip joints (Fig. 4–35). Note the two opposite forces that occur at the articulation between the fifth lumbar vertebra and the sacrum. In returning to the erect position, the pelvis is posteriorly rotated "under" the lumbar spine by concentric contraction of these same muscles.

Trunk forces also converge on the sacrum in the standing upright posture. The sacrum is oriented within the pelvis in a kyphotic and relatively flexed position. In upright standing the weight line courses down through the bodies of the lumbar vertebrae. The effect of this weight line through the lumbar vertebral bodies and onto the sacrum is to cause a flexion moment as the weight line converges on the superoanterior aspect of the vertebral body of the first sacral vertebra (Fig. 4–36).

Even more complex are the forces that are exerted on the sacroiliac joint owing to ground reaction forces. In these situations the innominate bone is mainly influenced by the transmission of forces through the femur, specifically how the femoral head compresses into or interacts with the acetabulum. However, the inability to precisely determine the exact type of movements that occur at the sacroiliac joints as a result of these forces is due to a lack of conclusive evidence as to the location of a horizontal axis around which the ilium can move on the sacrum. For example, Kapandji[47] shows a potential axis at Bonnaire's tubercle, which is a bony prominence between the cranial and caudal segments of the sacral articular surface, while Lavignolle and colleagues[51] calculate the horizontal axis of the sacroiliac joint to exist just posterior to the pubic symphysis.

Each of these two potential axes would yield quite different motions at the sacroiliac joint. In the first case (Fig. 4–37) more of a rotary motion of the ilium on the sacrum might occur, since the horizontal axis is through the articulating segments, that is, through the joint itself. The ilium would simply pivot around this axis on the sacrum. In the second case (Fig. 4–38) there would be more of a shearing stress, which would essentially be a type of upward

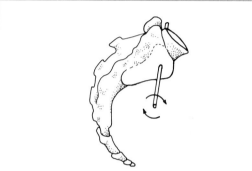

Figure 4–37. Sagittal view of the sacrum showing a potential axis at the apex of the cranial and caudal segments. A rotary moment is created about this transverse axis.

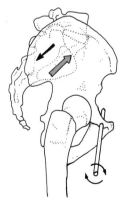

Figure 4–38. Sagittal view of the lumbopelvic region showing the second potential axis just posterior to the pubic symphysis. In this case the motion at the sacroiliac joint would be more of a shear force (see arrows) or sliding of the ilium on the sacrum rather than a true rotary moment, as hypothesized in Figure 4–37.

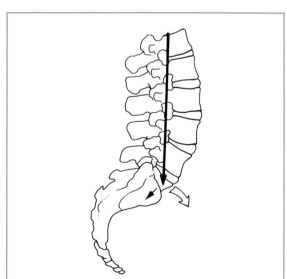

Figure 4–36. Sagittal view of the lumbar spine and sacrum. The vertical arrow indicates the trunk forces as they reach the sacrum, causing a flexion moment on the sacrum.

or downward "sliding" of the ilium on the sacrum, since the axis around which the bony segments now move is a great deal anterior to the sacroiliac joint.

Figure 4–39A shows the mechanics of the

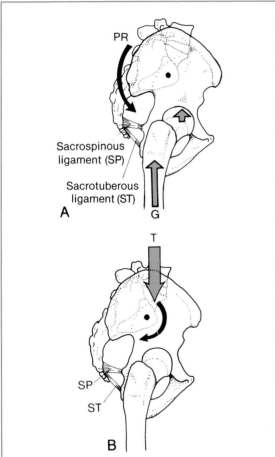

Figure 4–39. *A,* Sagittal view of the lumbopelvic region showing the ground force interacting with the ilia. The ground force (G) results in a posterior rotary force (PR) on the ilium. This is created by the anterior relation of the hip joint with respect to the sacroiliac joint. *B,* Sagittal view of the lumbopelvic region showing the reaction of the trunk force on the sacrum. The trunk force (T) produces a flexion moment on the sacrum. As compared with *A,* this motion is opposite, creating a natural screw home mechanism of the pelvis, which is stabilized by the sacrospinous and sacrotuberous ligaments.

joint with the assumption that the horizontal axis lies within the sacroiliac joint. The ground force (G), acting as the femur impacts and compresses into the acetabulum, causes a posterior rotary force on the ilium (PR). The reason for this posterior rotary force is that the region that the femoral head impacts on the acetabulum is anterior to the horizontal axis through the sacroiliac joint. This drives the roof of the acetabulum upward, which is a moment around a sacroiliac axis, causing a posterior rotation. The trunk force (T) produces an opposite motion on the sacrum, which is anterior rotation or flexion of the sacrum (Fig. 4–39B).[47] These forces result in the ilium and the sacrum rotating around the horizontal axis in opposite directions. The sacrotuberous and sacrospinous ligaments, by virtue of their attachments and orientation, offer a restraint to this motion. We consider the convergence of ground and trunk forces into this region with the resultant attenuation by the ligaments and the deformation of the cartilage owing to compression to be a type of "screw home" mechanism in the pelvis, which affords stability of the joint.

Although appreciable or excessive movement is possible in some people, especially multiparous, pregnant women and people with excessive connective tissue laxity, this is not the rule for the general population. Small, accommodating movements are most justifiable because of cartilage deformation as the sacroiliac joint surfaces engage and compress together during weight-bearing. However, rather than consider actual *movements* occurring, it appears more logical to consider the *moments* that are developed around various axes. These moments are generated by some of the most powerful muscles in the human body by virtue of their attachments to the pelvis, as well as ground and trunk forces. We consider it more logical to consider the resultant forces as a moment that the joint is rather well designed to accommodate rather than *movement* of the two bones. The cartilaginous surfaces compress and seat into each other as the trunk and ground forces are accepted and transferred by the lumbopelvic region during weight-bearing.

When there is a leg length discrepancy or any other frontal plane asymmetry, the pelvis

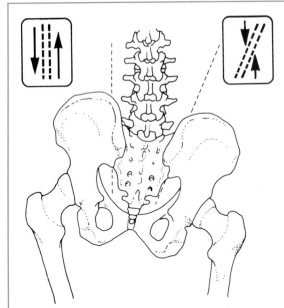

Figure 4–40. Frontal view of the lumbopelvic region showing a right frontal plane asymmetry (sacral base tilted down to the right). The upper right and upper left joint surfaces and arrows represent the forces to the left and right sacroiliac joints. The upper right box indicates a greater compressive force to the right sacroiliac joint as a result of changes in the joint surface, and the upper left box indicates a greater shear force to the left sacroiliac joint because of the more vertical relation of the joint surface in a right frontal plane asymmetry. The dotted lines indicate the sacroiliac joint surface.

is lower on one side. Ground reaction forces reach the lumbopelvic tissues differently, and the resultant forces are attenuated differently than in the symmetrical skeleton.[24,27,62,75,86] For example, with a short right leg the pelvis with its sacral base is tilted down to the right side (Fig. 4–40). This results in the right sacroiliac joint assuming a more relative horizontal position while the left sacroiliac joint is more vertical. Comparing the forces of the ilium on the sacrum with the symmetrical skeleton, more compressive force is applied to the right sacroiliac joint and more shear stress on the left. Because the sacral base, as it sits within the pelvis, is tilted down to the right, it also results in a side-bending motion at the lumbosacral joint.

Consequently compressive forces are placed on tissues on the concave side of the curve and tensile forces, on the convex side. If any of these forces exceed the tolerance of the tissues, there is a potential for tissue injury. Note how the frontal plane asymmetry potentially alters the mechanics at the sacroiliac joint, lumbosacral joint, and even the hip. For this reason it is extremely difficult to attempt to isolate one tissue at fault, but it is more logical to attempt to improve faulty mechanics that may contribute to the painful condition.

Therefore, as in any other joint, any position that takes the pelvic joints close to their end range, such as combined full forward and side bending, full backward and side bending, or moments applied to the hip joint that is already at extreme end range, renders the area vulnerable to injury. If the limits of sacroiliac joint motion are reached, and a force is then imparted through the lower extremities from below or through the upper extremities and trunk from above, there is a potential to sprain or strain the various supporting tissues.

PUBIC SYMPHYSIS

The pubic symphysis has come under close scrutiny as a potential cause of anterior pelvis and medial thigh pain since the early 1930s.[1,13] These authors recognized the vulnerability of this joint, especially with multiparous women, and described osseous changes to its structure.

The pubic symphysis is an amphiarthrodial joint in the anterior aspect of the pelvis that forms a fibrocartilaginous union between the two pubic bones. The pubis is the anterior part of the innominate bone. From its anteromedial body the superior ramus passes up and back to the acetabulum, while an inferior ramus passes back, down, and laterally to join the ischial ramus inferior to the obturator foramen.[99] The superior and inferior rami join anteriorly to form the body of the pubis, which has a symphysial (medial) surface that articulates with the contralateral pubis. The joint surface is lined with a thin layer of cartilage.[26] These joint surfaces are separated by a thick intrapubic fibrocartilaginous disc that is 3 to 5 mm wider anterior than posterior. The joint also includes a suprapubic ligament that attaches to the pubic tubercles and crests to cover the superior aspect of the joint. The anterior pubic symphysis blends with the aponeurosis of the rectus abdominis muscle, and the posterior aspect is connected by the posterior pubic ligament that joins with the inner abdominal fascia of the transversus abdominis muscle. The thick inferior pubic ligament or arcuate ligament forms an arch that spans both inferior rami and stabilizes the joint from compressive, shear, tensile, and rotary forces (Fig. 4–41).[26]

The structure of the symphysis is longer in the vertical direction in males, but the fibrocartilaginous disc is much wider in females.[26] The symphysis is used to determine skeletal age.[42,76] The investigators conclude that the symphysis pubis undergoes a variety of changes as a result of age, function, and, in females, the special hormonal influences of pregnancy and the mechanical trauma of parturition. This joint connects the two weight-bearing arches of the pelvis that together function to transfer and absorb the ground and trunk forces.

The pubic bone also provides attachment for

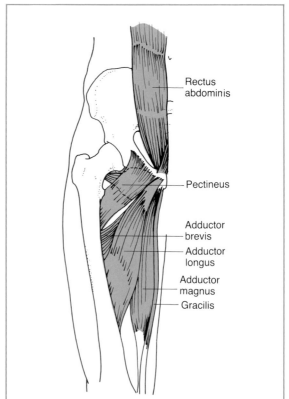

Figure 4–42. Anterior view of the pelvis and femur showing the attachment of the inferior medial thigh muscles and the rectus abdominis muscles as they attach into the superior and inferior ramus of the pubis.

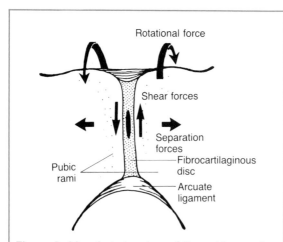

Figure 4–41. Anterior view of the pubic symphysis showing the superior and inferior ligamentous structures, and the forces that are generated to and must be counterbalanced by the anatomy of this articulation.

a number of different muscles. These muscles include the medial thigh muscles: the adductor longus, the adductor brevis, a portion of the adductor magnus, the gracilis, and the pectineus (Fig. 4–42). In addition, the rectus abdominis, the obturator internus and externus through their pubic portion of the obturator membrane, the pyramidalis, and the levator ani are attached. Many of these muscles, especially the medial thigh group, are large and quite capable of exerting significant forces to the pubis and, ultimately, the pelvic joints when the foot is fixed on the ground. These muscles play a major role in controlling the forces that are transferred into this region. The pubic symphysis resembles a bushing that permits tissue deformation and small translatory movements as a result of muscle, ground reaction, and trunk forces.

Numerous authors have studied the mechanics of this anterior pelvic joint, and have concluded that this amphiarthrodial joint has little movement, especially in men and nulliparous women.[15,26,50,68,76,91] In a more recent study parallel pins were inserted on either side of the pubic symphysis at the pubic tubercles on 15 subjects, all of whom were diagnosed with pelvic instability.[92] The findings revealed that the mean gap at the symphysis was 1 mm, and the forward-to-backward mean motion was 1.1 mm. Rotation was measured to average 0.5 degrees in both planes. The vertical translation varied among the population, but the mean distance was 2.5 mm. These findings support the concept that there is little movement available at the pubic symphysis for the clinician to quantify without sophisticated measuring devices. Like the sacroiliac joint, these small movements are representative of tissue deformation during force acceptance rather than actual joint excursion.

The pubic symphysis can be the site for pathological conditions, such as infectious and inflammatory diseases. The infectious diseases can be characteristic of intravenous drug users, and often involve pyogenic or tuberculous organisms.[81] The most common disease of the pubic symphysis is a self-limiting nonbacterial inflammation of the pubis that can be produced by pelvic surgery, childbirth, or trauma caused by work, play, or sport. The last is often attributed to repeated mechanical sprain or strain to the soft tissues that are attached to this region.[52,98]

Problems to the symphysis are not commonly seen in the clinic, but they can be recognized by the complaint of anterior pain often exacerbated by mechanical stresses of evaluation, such as posterior-to-anterior compression to the superior ramus of the pubis, resistance to contraction of the previously mentioned medial thigh muscles, and palpation. Tendinitis of the adductor longus or rectus abdominis can be easily mistaken for joint irritation because of the proximity of their attachments to the pubic symphysis. The problems related to treating the region are usually caused by the difficulty in stabilizing the area or controlling the resultant forces that reach it in order to allow for healing to occur.

THE HIP JOINT

Because movements of the hip joint ultimately transfer forces to the pelvis and lumbar regions, and the major muscle of the hip joint has attachments to these same regions, a brief review of the anatomy and mechanics is warranted. The hip joint is a multiaxial joint with the shape of a ball and socket. Because the complete surfaces of the femoral head and acetabulum are not in total contact with each other, nor are they true hemispheres, it is not a true ball-and-socket arrangement, but certainly approaches one.

The hip joint is very stable because of its design. Its architecture includes the acetabular labrum, which effectively deepens the socket. Because of the depth of the acetabulum, a vacuum effect is created when a distraction force is placed between the head of the femur and the acetabulum. The hip joint has the capability to move actively and passively in three planes. Approximate ranges of motion for hip joint mobility have been published elsewhere.[4] There are no accessory movements of the hip except for slight separation effected by strong traction.[99]

The hip joint capsule and the reinforcing ligaments provide a measure of joint stability as well as a check for motion. The ligamentous capsule is thicker anterosuperiorly, where maximal stress occurs, particularly in standing, while posteroinferiorly it is thin and loosely attached.[99] The capsular ligaments of the hip are divided into iliofemoral, ischiofemoral, and pubofemoral. These attachments are named for the areas of the innominate bone to which they are attached (Fig. 4–43). Anteriorly, the iliofemoral and pubofemoral ligaments converge to attach to the intertrochanteric line of the femur, whereas the ischiofemoral ligament originates from the ischium just posteroinferior to the acetabulum and spirals superolaterally behind the femoral neck to attach to the anterior aspect of the femur.

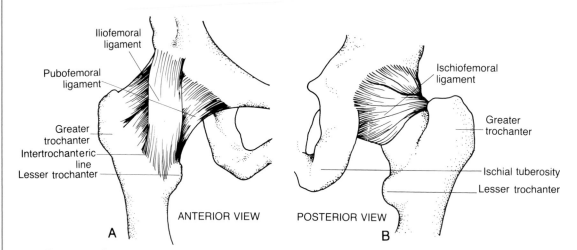

Figure 4–43. *A,* Anterior view of the right hip joint capsule showing the iliofemoral (ligament of Bigelow) and pubofemoral ligaments. Note the inferior and lateral direction of the anterior aspect of the hip joint capsule. *B,* Posterior view of the right hip joint indicating the fiber direction of the ischiofemoral ligament as it travels superiorly and laterally over the top of the femoral neck.

The close-packed position of the hip is full extension, with slight abduction and medial rotation.[99] Therefore, as this position is reached, the capsular ligaments of the hip become taut.[27,35,62,83] This position of the hip corresponds to the hip posture in standing. Although being at this close-packed position minimizes energy expenditure for upright posture, it also contributes to the fact that the hip joint has a higher incidence of degenerative joint disease than do joints that are not close-packed in standing, such as the ankle.[36] As the connective tissue limits of the hip joint capsular ligaments are reached, forces are subsequently transferred to the sacroiliac joints and then to the lumbar joints. Motion of the hip can thus influence pelvic and lumbar mechanics.

The hip is designed as a major weight-bearing joint with an articular cartilage–bony trabecular system that accepts large forces transferred through it.[33,43,45,77] The articular surfaces are reciprocally curved but not completely congruent. The acetabular articular surface is broader and thicker superiorly, where pressure of the body weight falls when in the erect, standing posture. The inferior surfaces of the femoral head do not articulate with the acetab-

ulum during loading and unloading. By contrast, the entire acetabulum is involved in weight-bearing.[16,32]

Contact and noncontact areas have been studied and both have been found to be involved in the degenerative process, suggesting that contact and a regular pattern of loading and unloading are necessary for normal joint lubrication and nutrition, which contribute to the overall health of the joint.[16,33,38] Degeneration patterns range from fibrillation of articular cartilage to osteophyte formation.[44,46]

The bony trabecular patterns of the femur and the pelvis dramatically illustrate the force transference system of the lumbopelvic region (Fig. 4–44). In the femur two trabecular patterns can be identified. These two trabecular patterns are oriented along compressive and tensile force lines. The acetabulum also reveals a trabecular pattern oriented along lines of stress.

Of perhaps greater interest to the clinician is the trabecular bone growth in response to forces traversing the hip, pelvis, sacrum, and lumbar spine. The trabecular pattern of these tissues reveals that the region is a true weight-bearing hub and works as an integral part of

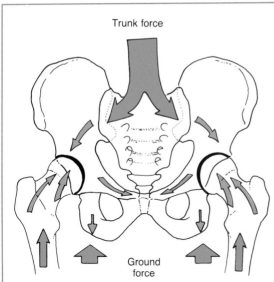

Figure 4–44. Anterior view of the bony structures of the lumbopelvic region. The arrows indicate the weight-bearing patterns of the lumbopelvic region with ground forces and trunk forces.

the lumbopelvic functional unit in order to transfer trunk and ground forces. The articulations of the lumbopelvic region are a linked system, and this linkage is emphasized by the trabecular pattern of the bones making up the linkage.

The femoral head can withstand 12 to 15 times body weight without destruction. The forces involved in single limb support standing on one leg, owing to the contraction of the hip abductor muscles and body weight, increase the load to 2.5 to 4 times body weight.[45] Running increases the load to approximately 5 times normal body weight.[45] The joint, therefore, is subject to such forces as body weight and muscle contraction.

Inherent in the design of the hip joint is an ability to deform and spread the loads over a larger surface area. This ability decreases the force per unit area and protects the articular cartilage from early degeneration.[31,60] Although compression is the major force imparted to the hip, it must also attenuate shear, bending, and torsion. The subchondral bone and trabecular pattern of the femur and the pelvis assist the articular cartilage in the transference of these forces.[43]

It is estimated that 10 per cent of people under age 30 have a degree of hip arthrosis, and this percentage rises to 89 per cent of those over age 65. The ratio of females to males showing degenerative changes is 3:2.[46] As these structural changes proceed, function can be assumed to be altered as well. However, it is not only movement at the hip joint itself that may be altered, but also the manner in which the hip joint transfers ground reaction forces to the pelvis and lumbar spine. The hip joint plays a major role in the proper transferral of forces through the axial skeleton. With respect to the lumbopelvic region, the hip plays an integral role and should be closely evaluated.

SUMMARY

We have defined the lumbopelvic unit as the articulations between L4 and L5, L5 and S1, the sacroiliac joint, the pubic symphysis, and hips. Each articulation has a unique design from which theories of function can be drawn. Some theories have withstood the rigor of experimental study, whereas others have yet to be proved. In addition, we have attempted to point out the interplay between not only these articulations, but also the soft tissues, including the musculature, that contribute to movement and weight-bearing by the lumbopelvic region. An understanding of these articulations will assist the clinician in the evaluation and treatment of mechanical disorders of this region. They are explored in the next chapters.

REFERENCES

1. Abramson D, Roberts SM, Wilson P: Relaxation of the pelvic joints in pregnancy. Gynecol Obstet (Sup) 58:595, 1934.
2. Adams MA, Hutton WC: The effect of posture on the role of the apophyseal joints in resisting intervertebral compressive forces. J Bone Joint Surg [Br] 62B:358, 1980.
3. Adams MA, Hutton WC: The relevance of torsion to the mechanical derangement of the lumbar spine. Spine 6:241, 1981.

4. American Academy of Orthopaedic Surgeons: Joint Motion: Method of Measuring and Recording. Chicago, American Academy of Orthopaedic Surgeons, 1965.

5. Bakland O, Hansen JH: The axial sacroiliac joint. Anat Clin 6:29, 1984.

6. Beal MC: The sacroiliac problem: Review of anatomy, mechanics and diagnosis. J Am Osteopath Assoc 81:667, 1982.

7. Bogduk N, Twomey LT: Clinical Anatomy of the Lumbar Spine. New York, Churchill Livingstone, 1987.

8. Borell U: The movements of the sacroiliac joints and their importance to changes in pelvic dimensions during parturition. Acta Gynecol Scand 36:42, 1957.

9. Bowan V, Cassidy JD: Macroscopic and microscopic anatomy of the sacroiliac joint from embryonic life until the eighth decade. Spine 6:620, 1981.

10. Bradford DS, Cooper KM, Oegema TR: Chymopapain, chemonucleolysis, and nucleus pulposus regeneration. J Bone Joint Surg (Am) 65A:1220, 1983.

11. Brickley-Parsons D, Glimcher MJ: Is the chemistry of collagen in intervertebral discs an expression of Wolff's law? Spine 9:148, 1984.

12. Brinckmann P: Injury of the annulus fibrosus and disc protrusions: An in vitro investigation of human lumbar discs. Spine 11:149, 1986.

13. Chamberlin WE: X-ray examination of the sacroiliac joints. Del Med J 4:195, 1932.

14. Colachis SD, Worden RE, Bechtol CO: Movement of the sacroiliac joint in the adult male: A preliminary report. Arch Phys Med Rehabil 44:490, 1963.

15. Coventry MB, Tapper EM: Pelvic instability. A consequence in removing ilial bone for grafting. J Bone Joint Surg (Am) 54A,10:83, 1972.

16. Day WH, Swanson SAV, Freeman MAR: Contact pressures in the loaded human cadaver hip. J Bone Joint Surg (Br) 57B:302, 1975.

17. Drerup B, Hierholzer E: Movement of the human pelvis and displacement of related anatomical landmarks on the body surface. J Biomech 20:971, 1987.

18. Dunlop RB, Adams MA, Hutton WC: Disc space narrowing and the lumbar facet joints. J Bone Joint Surg (Br) 66B:706, 1984.

19. Egund N: Movement in the sacroiliac joints demonstrated with roentgen stereophotogrammetry. Acta Radiol (Diagn) (Stockh) 19:833, 1978.

20. Erhard R, Bowling R, et al: The recognition and management of the pelvic components of low back and sciatic pain. Bulletin of Orthopedic Section. APTA 2:4, 1977.

21. Farfan HF: Mechanical Disorders of the Low Back. Philadelphia, Lea & Febiger, 1973.

22. Farfan HF, Cossette JW, Robertson GH, Wells RV: The effects of torsion on the lumbar intervertebral joints: The role of torsion in the production of disc degeneration. J Bone Joint Surg (Am) 52A:468, 1970.

23. Fraser DM: Postpartum backache: A preventable condition? Bulletin of Orthopedic Section, APTA 3:14, 1978.

24. Friberg O: Clinical symptoms and biomechanics of lumbar spine and hip joint in leg length inequality. Spine 8:643, 1983.

25. Frigerio NA: Movement of the sacroiliac joint. Clin Orthop 100:370, 1974.

26. Gamble JG, Simmons SC, Freedman M: The symphysis pubis. Clin Orthop 203:261, 1986.

27. Gofton JP: Osteoarthritis of the hip and leg length discrepancy. Can Med Assoc 104:791, 1971.

28. Golighty R: Pelvic arthropathy in pregnancy and the puerperium. Physiotherapy 68:216, 1982.

29. Gotfried Y, Bradford DS, Oegema TR: Facet joint changes after chemonucleolysis-induced disc space narrowing. Spine 11:944, 1986.

30. Gracovetsky S, Farfan H: The optimum spine. Spine 11:543, 1986.

31. Gradisar IA, Porterfield JA: Articular cartilage. Top Geriatr Rehab 4:1, 1989.

32. Greenwald AS, Haynes DW: Weight-bearing areas in the human hip joint. J Bone Joint Surg (Br) 54B:157, 1972.

33. Greenwald AS, O'Connor JJ: The transmission of load through the human hip joint. J Biomech 4:507, 1971.

34. Grieve E: Lumbo-pelvic rhythm and mechanical dysfunction of the sacroiliac joint. Physiotherapy 67:171, 1981.

35. Grieves GP: The hip. Physiotherapy 69:196, 1983.

36. Gruebel Lee DM: Disorders of the Hip. Philadelphia, JB Lippincott, 1983, p. 1.

37. Hampton D, Laros G, McCarron R, Franks D: Healing potential of the annulus fibrosus. Spine 14:398, 1989.

38. Harrison MHM, Schajowicz F, Truetta J: Osteoarthritis of the hip: A study of the nature and evolution of the disease. J Bone Joint Surg (Br) 35B:77, 1953.

39. Hishaw TL: Corpus luteum hormone: Experimental relaxation of pelvic ligaments of guinea pig. Physiol Zool 2:59, 1929.

40. Hoppenfeld S: Physical Examination of the Spine and Extremities. New York, Appleton-Century-Crofts, 1976.

41. Horton GW: Further observations on the elastic mechanism of the intervertebral disc. J Bone Joint Surg (Br) 40B:552, 1958.

42. Jackes MK: Pubic symphysis age distribution. Am J Phys Anthropol 68:281, 1985.

43. Jacob HAV, Huggler AH, Dietschi C, Schreiber A: Mechanical function of subchondral bone as experimentally determined on the acetabulum of the human pelvis. J Biomech 9:625, 1976.

44. Jeffery AK: Osteophyte and the osteoarthritic femoral head. J Bone Joint Surg (Br) 57B:314, 1975.

45. Johnston R: Mechanical considerations of the hip joint. Arch Surg 107:411, 1973.

46. Jorring K: Osteoarthritis of the hip. Acta Orthop Scand 51:523, 1980.

47. Kapandji IA: The Physiology of the Joints, vol 3. Edinburgh, Churchill Livingstone, 1974.

48. Klein J, Hukins D: X-ray diffraction demonstrates re-orientation of collagen fibres in the annulus fibrosus during compression of the intervertebral disc. Biochim Biophys Acta 717:61, 1982.

49. Klein J, Hukins D: Collagen fibre orientation in the annulus fibrosus of intervertebral disc during bending and torsion measured by X-ray diffraction. Biochim Biophys Acta 719:98, 1982.

50. Laban MN, Meerschaert JR, Taylor RS, Tabor HD: Symphyseal and sacroiliac joint pain associated with pubic symphyseal instability. Arch Phys Med Rehab 59:470, 1978.

51. Lavignolle B, Vital JM, Senegas J, et al: An approach to the functional anatomy of the sacroiliac joints in vivo. Anat Clin 5:169, 1983.

52. Le Jeune JJ, Rochcongar P, Vazelle F, et al: Pubic pain syndrome in sportsmen: Comparison of radiographic and scintigraphic findings. Eur J Nucl Med 9:250, 1984.

53. Luk KDK, Ho HC, Leong JCY: The iliolumbar ligament: A study of its anatomy, development and clinical significance. J Bone Joint Surg (Br) 68B:197, 1986.

54. Lumsden RM, Morris JM: An in vivo study of axial rotation and immobilization at the lumbosacral joint. J Bone Joint Surg [Am] 50:1591, 1968.

55. Maitland GD: Vertebral Manipulation, 3rd ed. London, Butterworth Publishers, 1973.

56. Malinsky J: The ontogenetic development of nerve terminations in the intervertebral discs of man. Acta Anat (Basel) 38:96, 1959.

57. Markolf KL, Morris JM: The structural components of the intervertebral disc. J Bone Joint Surg [Am] 56A:675, 1974.

58. McCarron RF, Wimpee MW, Hudkins PG, Laros GS: The inflammatory effect of the nucleus pulposus: A possible element in the pathogenesis of lowback pain. Spine 12:760, 1987.

59. McKenzie RA: Mechanical Diagnosis and Therapy of the Lumbar Spine. Waikanae, New Zealand, Spinal Publications, 1981.

60. Meachim G: Effect of age on the thickness of adult articular cartilage at the shoulder joint. Ann Rheum Dis 30:43, 1971.

61. Meachim G, Stockwell RA: The matrix. In Freeman MAR (ed): Adult Articular Cartilage. New York, Grune & Stratton, 1972, pp. 1–50.

62. Mellin G: Correlations of hip mobility with degree of back pain and lumbar spinal mobility in chronic low-back pain patients. Spine 13:668, 1988.

63. Mennell JM: Diagnosis and Treatment Using Manipulative Techniques: Joint Pain. Boston, Little, Brown, 1964.

64. Mitchell FL: An Evaluation and Treatment Manual of Osteopathic Muscle Energy Procedures. Valley Park, Mo, Mitchell, Moran & Pruzzo, 1979.

65. Mooney V, Robertson J: The facet syndrome. Clin Orthop 115:149, 1976.

66. Nachemson A: Towards a better understanding of low-back pain: A review of the mechanics of the lumbar disc. Rheumatol Rehab 14:129, 1975.

67. Nachemson A, Morris JM: In vivo measurements of intradiscal pressure. J Bone Joint Surg 46:1077, 1964.

68. Olerud S, Greusten S: Chronic symphysiolysis. A case report. J Bone Joint Surg (Am) 56A:799, 1974.

69. Panjabi MM, Krag MH, Chung TQ: Effects of disc injury on mechanical behavior of the human spine. Spine 9:707, 1984.

70. Paquin JD, van der Rest M, Marie PJ, et al: Biochemical and morphologic studies of cartilage from the adult human sacroiliac joint. Arthritis Rheum 26:887, 1983.

71. Paris S: Anatomy as related to function and pain. Orthop Clin North Am 14:475, 1983.

72. Pearcy MJ, Tibrewal SB: Lumbar intervertebral disc and ligament deformations measured in vivo. Clin Orthop 191:281, 1984.

73. Pitkin HD, Pheasant HC, et al: Sacrarthrogenetic telalgia. J Bone Joint Surg [Am] 18:111, 1936.

74. Porterfield JA: Dynamic stabilization of the trunk. J Orthop Sports Phys Ther 6:271, 1985.

75. Porterfield JA, DeRosa CP: The sacroiliac joint. In Gould JA (ed): Orthopedic and Sports Physical Therapy, 2nd ed. St. Louis, CV Mosby, 1990, p. 553.

76. Putschar WGJ: The structure of the human symphysis pubis with special consideration of parturition and its sequelae. Am J Anthrop 45:589, 1931.

77. Ramamurti C: In Finker R (ed): Orthopaedics in Primary Care. Baltimore, Williams & Wilkins, 1979, p. 1.

78. Roberts S, Menage J, Urban JPG: Biochemical and structural properties of the cartilage end-plate and its relation to the intervertebral disc. Spine 14:166, 1989.

79. Sashin D: A critical analysis of the anatomy and the pathological changes of the SI joints. J Bone Joint Surg [Am] 12:891, 1930.

80. Schunke GB: The anatomy and the development of the sacroiliac joint and their relation to the movements of the sacrum. Acta Anat (Basel) 23:80, 1955.

81. Sequeria W, Jones E, Seigel ME, et al: Pyogenic infections of the pubic symphysis. Ann Intern Med 96:604, 1982.

82. Solonen KA: The sacroiliac joint in light of anatomical, roentgenological, and clinical studies. Acta Orthop Scand [Suppl] 27:1, 1957.

83. Steindler A: Kinesiology of the Human Body Under Normal and Pathological Conditions. Springfield, Ill, Charles C Thomas, 1955.

84. Stoddard A: Manual of Osteopathic Technique. London, Hutchinson & Co., 1959, p. 211.

85. Sturesson B, Selvik G, Uden A: Movements of the sacroiliac joints: A roentgen stereophotogrammetric analysis. Spine 14:162, 1989.

86. Subotnick S: Podiatric Sports Medicine. Mount Kisco, NY, Futura Publishing Co, 1975.

87. Taylor JR, Twomey LT: Age changes in lumbar zygapophyseal joints: Observation on structure and function. Spine 11:739, 1986.

88. Tesh KM, Dunn JS, Evans JH: The abdominal muscles and vertebral stability. Spine 12:501, 1987.

89. Twomey LT, Taylor JR: Sagittal movements of the human lumbar vertebral column: A quantitative study of the role of the posterior vertebral elements. Arch Phys Med Rehabil 64:322, 1983.

90. Virgin W: Experimental investigation into the physical properties of the intervertebral disc. J Bone Joint Surg (Br) 33B:607, 1951.

91. Vix VA, Ryu CY: The adult symphysis pubis: Normal and abnormal. Am J Roentgenol 112:517, 1971.

92. Walheim GG, Olerud S, Ridde T: Mobility of the pubic symphysis. Measurements by an electromechanical method. Acta Orthop Scand 55:203, 1984.

93. Walker JM: Age-related differences in the human sacroiliac joint: A histological study; implications for therapy. J Orthop Sports Phys Ther 7:325, 1986.

94. Weisl H: Movements of the sacroiliac joint. Acta Anat (Basel) 23:80, 1955.

95. Weisl H: The articular surfaces of the sacroiliac joint and their relation to the movement of the sacrum. Acta Anat (Basel) 22:1, 1954.

96. Weiss M, Nagelschmidt M, Struck H: Relaxin and collagen metabolism. Horm Metab Res 11:408, 1979.

97. White AA, Panjabi MM: Clinical Biomechanics of the Spine. Philadelphia, JB Lippincott, 1978.

98. Wiley JJ: Traumatic osteitis pubis: The gracilis syndrome. Am J Sports Med 11:360, 1983.

99. Williams PL, Warwick R, Dyson M, Bannister LH: Gray's Anatomy. London, Churchill Livingstone, 1989.

100. Wyke B: Neurological aspects of low back pain. In Jayson M (ed): The Lumbar Spine and Back Pain. Grune and Stratton, New York, 1976, p. 173.

101. Wyke B: The neurology of low back pain. In Jayson M (ed): The Lumbar Spine and Back Pain, 2nd ed. Tunbridge Wells, Pitman Medical, 1980, p. 265.

102. Yasuma T, Makino E, Saito S, Inui M: Histological development of intervertebral disc herniation. J Bone Joint Surg (Am) 68A:1066, 1986.

103. Zarins B: Soft tissue injury and repair—biomechanical aspects. Int J Sports Med 3:9, 1982.

5

FUNCTIONAL ASSESSMENT OF THE LUMBOPELVIC REGION

A point that has been stressed throughout the text thus far is that it is difficult to isolate the exact tissue that is injured in most low back disorders. It has also been mentioned that low back pain can be referred from other structures, including the pelvic and abdominal viscera. Therefore, a complete evaluation of the patient who is complaining of low back pain requires background knowledge of pathology in order that the clinician can begin to sort the mechanical disorders from those that are nonmechanical. It is beyond the scope of this text to present details of pathology. Instead, this chapter focuses on the important component of the evaluation process called the *functional assessment*. As the name implies, this evaluation process emphasizes the analysis of function. Varying stresses and movements are intro-duced into the lumbopelvic region in order to assess the response. With a strong understanding of the purpose and rationale behind functional assessment, the clinician can then add specific questions or tests that might be indicated in order to rule out low back pain from nonmechanical causes.

In order to understand the implications of mechanical and inflammatory conditions of the lumbosacral nerve roots, the neurologic screening examination to assess nerve root involvement was discussed in Chapter 2. This allowed the neurologic examination to be viewed in the context of the relevant neuroanatomy and neurophysiology. Because the examination is not repeated here, the reader is encouraged to incorporate the neurologic examination into the functional assessment.

The key to proper functional assessment of the low back–injured patient is determining the position(s) that exacerbate the familiar symptoms that motivated the patient to seek professional help. Reproducing the pain syndrome is the basis for functional assessment. Because of the inherent difficulties in isolating the exact injured tissue involved, this evaluation concept focuses on the forces generated with changes in body position and subsequent muscle contraction that converge in the lumbopelvic region and exacerbate symptoms. It can then be deduced which forces exceed the tissue's tolerance or adaptability, and therefore mechanically and/or chemically stimulate the nociceptive system to give rise to the perception of pain.

Many tests have been devised to evaluate the function and the painful syndrome of the low back region.[6] One hypothesis often entertained contends that the articulations of the low back are the main source of the syndrome, and that repositioning or mobilizing joint processes should be the primary goal of rehabilitation. This is not to say that this approach is not warranted in some instances; however, it does not appear to represent the complete answer in the long-term successful management of low back pain. Additionally, many evaluation tests implemented in the lumbopelvic region are often not based on the physical sciences, such as anatomy, physiology, and kinesiology. Although neural and discal tissues unique to this region do lend to its complexity, the clinician should continue to respect basic properties of the primary body tissues, including bone, muscle, and connective tissue, as they will remain consistent whether constituting the knee or the back.

Other approaches to evaluation of low back pain are based on the notion that the tissue of origin can be accurately and specifically identified. Not only is the determination of the exact tissue involved in the painful syndrome difficult, but even with current technology, the findings do not always correlate with the clinical symptoms.[8,14,16,21,25,29] With the emergence of new technology, such as computed tomography and magnetic resonance imaging, the structures within and surrounding the spinal canal, including soft tissues, can be better vis-

ualized. Although these diagnostic tests are certainly of significant value, it is essential that the findings are correlated with and reaffirmed by a functional clinical impression to determine an appropriate treatment plan and maximize the patient's potential for recovery. It is recognized that low back pain and disability do not progressively increase with age, nor do they correlate with the natural degenerative changes of the intervertebral disc.[11,30] It is also understood that treatment that involves increased activity promotes muscle and bone growth[2,22,26] and minimizes sensitivity to pain.[17]

Therefore, the clinician should remember that (a) as in any region of the body, an isolated lesion is uncommon because it is often associated with an injury process or changes in related tissues; (b) the composition of bone, muscle, and connective tissue and their physiologic properties are consistent in the back, as in any other area; and (c) basing the evaluation system on one specific aspect or tissue of the lumbopelvic region, without considering the mechanism of injury and forces that reproduce familiar symptoms, may hinder the opportunity for achieving long-term results. The goal of a functional assessment is to take the subjective and objective findings and correlate them to the circumstances of the injury or onset to determine the following:

1. The positions of weight-bearing posture of the lumbopelvic region that produce the patient's pain complaint

2. The pattern of the painful syndrome

3. The inflammatory status or state of the injured tissue(s)

4. The appropriate treatment plan to be implemented

This assessment system is designed to assist the clinician in the determination of the antigravity forces that increase the patient's pain. This must first be established in the standing position and then *substantiated* in the prone, supine, and sitting positions. In order to be successful at this approach, the clinician must gain a three-dimensional understanding of the static and dynamic anatomy of this region. This entails visualizing the forces generated throughout the tissues of the low back, pelvis, and hips from superior to inferior, inferior to superior, and in all three planes of movement as the varying positional changes of the functional assessment proceed. The examiner should also be able to judge the irritability of the injured tissue(s) by the amount of stress required to evoke a given painful response from the patient. This procedure is designed to give the examiner a way to cross check the region by allowing him or her to generate movements and forces into the lumbopelvic region and thus assess the *matches*, or similarities, within the functional assessment. If the examiner can effectively use this assessment system to identify the destructive and nondestructive ranges of motion, an appropriate treatment plan can be developed.

The following functional assessment scheme is used to evaluate mechanical low back pain syndromes. It should be recognized that many testing positions can be performed in the evaluation process. If a test maneuver is not described within the confines of this text, the reader should not conclude that it has no worth in the assessment process. It does not matter what stresses are used to provoke a familiar symptom as long as the clinician can identify the intensity and direction of the force used and the interrelation of the force of the test and the mechanics of the painful syndrome.

This chapter aims to help identify mechanical low back pain. If the clinician is unable to correlate or *match* the findings in the various test positions, then the source of the syndrome may be nonmechanical. The clinician should then be suspicious of the other causes of low back pain, and further diagnostics are indicated.

HISTORY

The first part of any examination is the history. It should be structured so that it provides a mechanism for the clinician and patient to reach a common understanding as to the nature of the problem. This is the first step in getting the patient to recognize that he or she is an integral part of a successful management program.

It is important that the clinician ask questions that will elicit information to help discern whether the patient may be having pain of a nonmechanical source, such as abdominal or pelvic visceral pathology. This information also will help to determine whether referral for further evaluation is indicated. Complaints such as fever, night pain, metabolic disease, and bowel or bladder disturbances and factors such as medications currently used and a past medical history of cancer indicate the importance of knowledge of pathology in order that appropriate referral can be made if necessary. In addition, the patient's occupation and a clear idea by the clinician of the demands of that job are also important. With recognition of these important points, what follows is the detailed analysis of the major components of the history used for the functional assessment of mechanical disorders of the lumbopelvic region.

Six important components of information should be obtained (Table 5–1): (1) the duration of pain—how long the patient has had it; (2) the position of injury; (3) the pain pattern (location, intensity, frequency, and duration); (4) number and duration of pain episodes since onset; (5) positions or activities that aggravate the pain; and (6) the patient's impression as to the source of the problem. This information can be arrived at in a variety of ways, but to finish the history without at least this basic information minimizes the chances to envision the forces of injury that probably occurred and are perhaps representing the source of the problem.

The patient is first asked to complete a questionnaire that provides the clinician with information concerning the patient's name, age, weight, height, employment status, and existing medical problems and the quantification from 0 to 10 of the patient's perception of the

TABLE 5–1. Information Gained from the History

1. Pain duration
2. Position of the body at injury
3. Pain pattern
4. Number and duration of pain episodes since onset
5. Positions and movements of symptom reproduction
6. Patient's perception of the problem

intensity of pain and the limitation of activity (Table 5–2). The patient is also instructed to indicate the location of his pain on an illustration drawn on the questionnaire. The information gleaned from the questionnaire is invaluable, and assisting the patient in completing the questionnaire can provide the starting point of the history. Once the questionnaire is satisfactorily completed, the examiner begins by asking the following questions.

How Long Have You Had Low Back Pain?

Determining the duration of the painful syndrome is important in order to establish length of time that the body has had to adapt to the injury. If the patient has recently experienced the initial bout of the injury, then the process of neuromuscular and connective tissue adaptation is probably minimal. On the other hand, consider the patient who experienced the initial bout of injury 7 years ago and has had five exacerbations of the same pain. Depending on the body's ability to functionally adapt, significant adaptations may have resulted, causing a decreased pain threshold. Utilizing two graphs that compare the intensity versus time for the entire history and for a 24-hour period is important for both the patient and the clinician to visualize the pain pattern (Fig. 5–1).

TABLE 5–2. Intake Questionnaire

Name: _____ Date: _____

Age: _____ Sex: _____ Height: _____ Weight: _____

Employer: _____

    Address: _____

    _____

    Phone: (____) _____

    Supervisor's Name: _____

List existing medical problems other than your musculoskeletal pain.

_____

_____

PAIN SCALE:

If 0 equals no pain and 10 equals the worst pain that you have experienced with this problem, please circle your present level of pain:

0   1   2   3   4   5   6   7   8   9   10

ACTIVITY SCALE:

If 0 equals bed rest or no activity, and 10 equals what you determine to be normal activity, please circle your current level of activity:

0   1   2   3   4   5   6   7   8   9   10

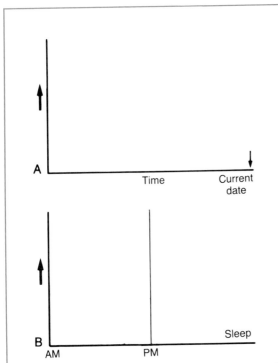

Figure 5–1. *A,* Graph showing the intensity of pain along the vertical and the time along the horizontal. This allows the clinician to take a history with respect to intensity, frequency, and duration of the pain pattern. This simple way of graphically outlining the patient's history is an important tool not only to allow the patient to visualize his history, but also to have something tangible that the patient and the clinician can relate to. *B,* Graph showing the intensity of pain along the vertical from morning to evening or a 24-hour period on the horizontal, allowing the clinician and patient to agree on a daily painful period.

What Position Were You in When You Were Initially Injured?

Recreating the position of injury, if possible, provides information regarding the biomechanics involved in the painful syndrome. From this information the clinician can make a judgment as to the compression, tension, torsion, and shear forces involved in the position

of injury, and can speculate as to the extent of the damage. If the patient cannot identify a specific position of injury, then the questioning should be directed toward determining the extent of work and extracurricular activity the patient was experiencing at or previous to the time of initial onset. It is not uncommon for the patient to have difficulty in identifying a specific position of injury, but the clinician should gain an appreciation as to the extent and level of activity so that some judgment can be made. Once the judgment of the biomechanics of the injury has been made, the clinician needs to establish the location of the injury.

Show Me Where You Have Pain

A drawing of a posterior view of the skeleton is printed on the same side of the form as the graphs so that the clinician can indicate which part of the back or lower quarter is symptomatic (Fig. 5–2). This information should be immediately compared with the drawing done by the patient on the intake questionnaire. If the drawings coincide, then the history continues. If the drawings are noticeably different, then time should be taken to clarify the location of the symptom(s). The patient is asked to show the clinician on the drawing and to demonstrate on himself or herself exactly where the pain is located, and a reference is established for both the clinician and the patient for future comparison.

Now that the duration and location of the pain and the mechanics of the injury have been determined, the parameters of the pain pattern (intensity and frequency) must be established.

How Many Episodes of the Pain Have You Had Since the Onset and How Long Has Each Lasted?

The frequency and intensity can easily be recorded on the graphs. Figure 5–3A is a graphic representation of a case study. In this

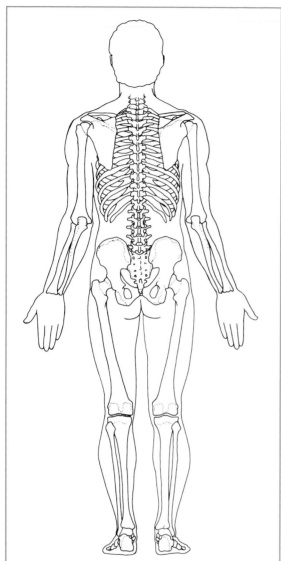

Figure 5–2. Posterior view of the skeleton. This allows the patient and clinician to indicate the painful site. The drawing can be placed on the same sheet as the graphs, which permits the clinician to complete the history-taking process in a visual manner.

back in the same location to the same level of pain intensity 6 months later. This time the intensity completely diminished but took 4 to 6 weeks. Two months ago the patient reinjured his back at work, and the pain intensity has been fluctuating between a 7 and a 10. The patient then decided to seek professional help and enters the clinician's office with pain at the intensity of 7.

A second graph relates intensity to a 24-hour period. Figure 5–3B shows that the patient awakes with stiffness and mild pain. As the day progresses the pain decreases but then begins to intensify by the end of the day. The patient has no difficulty sleeping. This pattern suggests that the patient awakens with swelling of the injured tissue(s), which stimulates the receptor system, giving rise to pain and stiffness. This swelling is due to the vasodilation that occurs during the initial stages of healing as well as to fluid stasis.[1,12,31]

As movement begins the mechanoreceptors are stimulated to help modulate pain, and the pressures generated by muscle contraction help to decrease fluid stasis. By the end of the day, however, the injured tissue has been subjected to forces that exceed its physical tolerance, and the pain begins to increase.

If the morning is the best time of the day, and the pain increases after periods of weight-bearing and movement, then that person's anti-gravity joint and muscle mechanics are unable to keep the tissues in an invulnerable range. Invulnerable range refers to that range of motion that is within the tissues' tolerance to a given intensity of forces that does not cause further damage (see Chapter 1, Fig. 1–7). This group of patients will probably respond quite well to those rehabilitative activities that are designed to improve weight-bearing mechanics during the time the patient is counterbalancing the forces of gravity. Many mechanical low back pain patients describe an increase in pain at the end of the day, which probably represents the inability to maintain the invulnerable range of the injured tissues. The continuous active and passive forces generated to the musculoskeletal tissues during the activities of daily living result in increased pain by the end of the day. On the other hand, rest and unloading these tissues help to decrease pain.

example the patient states that he sustained a lifting injury 3 years ago. That pain remained for 3 weeks and then gradually and completely resolved. However, the patient reinjured his

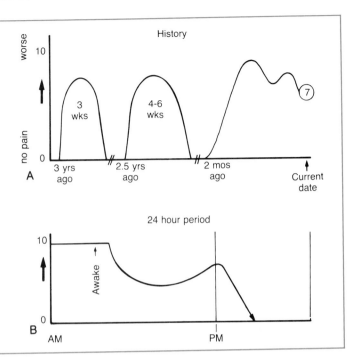

Figure 5–3. *A,* Graph showing an example of a patient who had an injury 3 years ago that lasted for 3 weeks, experienced the same injury 2½ years ago that lasted for 4 to 6 weeks, and then reinjured himself 2 months ago and has been fluctuating between 7 and 10 for that amount of time. The current rate is 7 on a 10 scale. *B,* Twenty-four-hour chart showing that the patient awoke with pain and stiffness that gradually declined as the day progressed, but then had increased pain at the end of the day. There was no complaint of pain in the evening that altered the patient's sleeping pattern.

What Position(s) and Activities Increase Your Pain?

This question directs the patient's thinking toward his activities of daily living. It is important for the patient to scrutinize these activities because ultimately the patient must recognize the relation between those activities and the continuation of the painful syndrome. If the patient cannot clearly answer this question, then the clinician should explain that a goal of the assessment is to clarify this answer so that the destructive movements during the time away from the clinic can be decreased.

After this discussion the patient reviews the graphs and is asked if this accurately represents his problem. Many patients make subtle changes on the graphs to more accurately describe the intensity or the time. This is encouraged because once the patient has made an effort to make the graph correct, he is taking an active role in understanding his problem. The clinician can also begin to make a judgment

about the interest of his patient with respect to his motivation to recovery.

The graphs are important from another perspective. The goal of treatment is to minimize the intensity of pain and extend the duration of the pain-free periods. Evidence of reaching this goal can be read from the graphs, since they represent a tangible record of the patient's pain pattern. Establishing this vehicle for communication provides the clinician and patient with a mechanism to evaluate the treatment's effectiveness.

The patient must learn to recognize that success in the management of low back pain syndromes represents a small change in the intensity, frequency, or duration of pain. If the patient does not experience change after a reasonable number of treatments, then reevaluation is indicated to redirect the treatment process.

The sixth category of questions asked during a history deals with directing the patient's attention to the fact that his problem is his responsibility, not the clinician's. Additionally, the information provided by the patient gives the clinician a better idea of the patient's perception of the problem.

What Do You Think Is the Cause of Your Back Pain?

Most patients answer this question with "I don't know." The clinician should encourage some form of answer. This can be done by making a statement such as, "You must have some impression as to what is happening in your back. Does it feel like something is grinding, or squeezing, or slipping, or . . . ?" The clinician should then pause and allow the patient to finish the thought. Although it is recognized that this can be construed as influencing the patient's thoughts, we believe that it is an important bit of information because the intent is to gain a clear conception as to how the patient views his problem. Most patients explain their impression in their own words. If a patient is unable to carry out this thought, the clinician must judge whether the patient is unable to express himself, or whether the patient is unwilling to divulge the needed information. The clinician, by this time, should be able to judge whether the patient is interested in obtaining a recovery.

Other data that should be obtained during the history are (a) any previous medical problems that may relate to the current complaint of pain and (b) what previous treatment, including diagnostic tests, was performed.

There are many methods of obtaining a good history, and the clinician should develop his or her own method of gathering at least the aforementioned six points of information. The questioning should be done in a logical progression, so that the patient can follow the sequencing of the history. If the patient is able to follow the line of questioning and relate one question to another, then he will be better able to assist the clinician in implementing a successful treatment sequence.

These are some of the important details of the history. If further questions regarding other medical problems are indicated, they should be addressed. On completion of the history, the objective examination begins by proceeding with the examination from the standing position.

STANDING EXAMINATION

Table 5–3 outlines the sequence of the standing examination.

Observation

While the patient stands, the examiner views the patient's posterior aspect (Fig. 5–4). From this position the examiner is looking for any asymmetries or deviations from the expected norm, such as side shifting, listing, or the inability to bear weight on one side compared with the other. The examiner should begin at the occiput and observe the position of the head, shoulders, arms, and scapulae. It is important to note that considerable variations and adaptations occur in the upper portion of the body owing to lumbopelvic disorders. For example, a person who has a frontal plane asymmetry at the pelvis may or may not have uneven shoulders. The upper quarter does not always match the lower quarter in the standing position; this should not be ignored, but rather observed and noted. If both quarters match, then the clinical picture becomes clearer.

TABLE 5–3. Standing Examination

A. Inspection
   1. Sagittal plane
   2. Frontal plane
B. Gait analysis
C. Structural examination
   1. Palpate level and position
      a. Iliac crest
      b. PSIS
      c. ASIS
      d. Greater trochanters
   2. Frontal plane correction, if indicated
D. Gross movement testing (GMT) (Familiar symptom reproduction)
   1. Active forward bending
   2. Active backward bending
   3. Guided movement with overpressure
      a. Forward bending
      b. Forward bending–side bending
      c. Backward bending
      d. Backward bending–side bending
      e. Any combination of FB, BB, SB, and rotation that reproduces the familiar symptoms
E. Neurologic screening (Chapter 2)

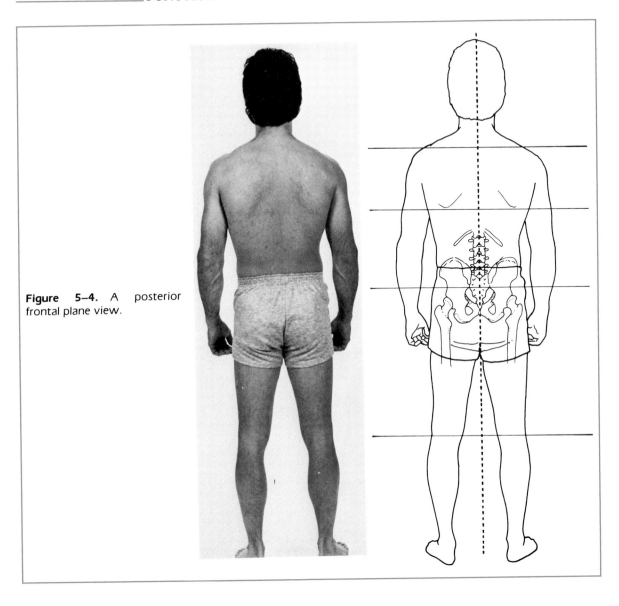

Figure 5–4. A posterior frontal plane view.

The inspection continues by following the spine from the upper thoracic region to the sacrum. If scoliosis is suspected, it can be verified by the forward bend test to determine the presence of a rib hump. The contours and the symmetry of the waist angles (i.e., the angles that the skin fold makes above the iliac crest) should be noted.

The pelvis is then observed. Attention should be given to the orientation of the pelvis in the three cardinal planes, especially the frontal plane from the posterior view. This can be seen by looking at the soft-tissue masses at the superior aspect of the ilium. Because this is an area of adipose tissue storage, it may not yield any relevant clinical information. If the patient is relatively lean, the examiner can easily observe the antigravity position of the pelvis in the frontal and sagittal positions. The inspection continues down the back of both thighs to the Achilles tendons. These tendons should be vertical. If they are asymmetrical or both bow in, then the calcaneus is likely to be excessively everted and an evaluation of the foot would be indicated.[15] It is important to understand the relation between foot mechanics and the alteration of the normal weight-bearing pattern as the ground forces reach the lumbopelvic tissues.

An analysis of gait can provide useful information regarding the weight-bearing capabilities of the musculoskeletal system.[15,20] For example, excessive pronation throughout the stance phase results in increased extension stress to the lumbar spine because of the obligatory downward tilt of the pelvis. Excessive supination of the foot throughout the stance phase potentially results in a decrease in the attenuation of ground forces, which may increase stress to the lumbopelvic region.

Structural Examination

There are numerous ways to carry out a structural examination of the lumbopelvic region. However, the clinician should develop a routine of evaluating every lumbopelvic prob-

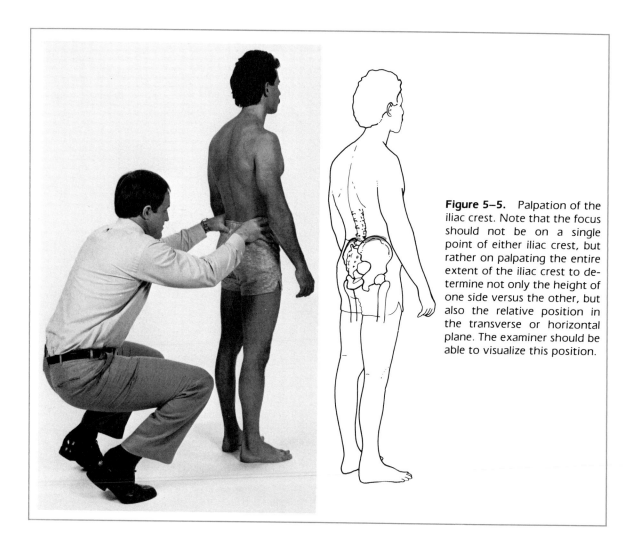

Figure 5–5. Palpation of the iliac crest. Note that the focus should not be on a single point of either iliac crest, but rather on palpating the entire extent of the iliac crest to determine not only the height of one side versus the other, but also the relative position in the transverse or horizontal plane. The examiner should be able to visualize this position.

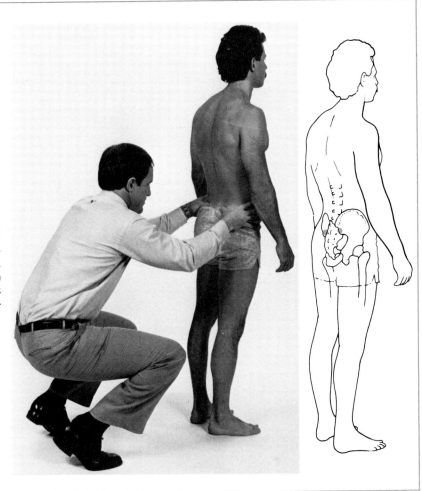

Figure 5–6. The second palpation point is the posterior superior iliac spine (PSIS). The examiner should strive to place the thumb inferior to the PSIS in the "shelf" as the sacrum meets the ilium. This is the most important point in the pelvis because the ledge is the most distinguishable palpation point.

lem the same way. By collecting data in a consistent manner, comparisons can be made among many patients.

The standing weight-bearing examination is one of the most important parts of the overall assessment. Most mechanical low back pain problems are exacerbated by upright positions and movement patterns and relieved by recumbency. The manner in which forces reach tissues is different when the person is standing than when he is supine or prone. It is much easier for a person to place the injured low back structures into nonpainful positions when the forces of weight-bearing are removed.

Four bony landmarks are assessed: the iliac crest, the posterior superior iliac spines (PSIS), the anterior superior iliac spine (ASIS), and the greater trochanter. The goal with these palpations is to visualize a three-dimensional picture of the position of the pelvis. The complete extent of the iliac crest is palpated in order to provide the clinician with information to be used for assessing pelvic position. This assessment is achieved by comparing the bony elements of both sides (Fig. 5–5).

The PSIS are then palpated by starting caudal to their location and moving the thumbs upward in an attempt to hook under these bony prominences (Fig. 5–6). The "dimples" are surface landmarks that approximate these bony prominences. If the examiner finds these landmarks difficult to locate, he or she can start at the apex of the sacrum and palpate superiorly and laterally along the surface of the sacrum until the edge of the ilium is felt. The large processes palpated in this region are the PSIS. Either technique—hooking under the PSIS or following the sacrum superiorly and laterally—helps to place the two palpating thumbs in relatively the same position on the right and left PSIS. This palpation gives the clinician the perception of the frontal plane position of the pelvis, which is the first step in determining the position of the sacral base.

The next palpation point is the ASIS and the iliac crests (Fig. 5–7). The ASIS is a large bony prominence, and it is difficult to palpate a single symmetrical identifying point. Therefore,

the complete extent of the iliac crest should again be palpated in conjunction with the ASIS. The frontal plane position and the symmetry should be noted.

We suggest that the clinician stop now and assess the findings from these three palpations. These bony landmarks of the pelvis give the clinician a reasonable three-dimensional picture of the pelvis with its accompanying sacral base. The position of the sacral base is important because it helps the examiner to visualize the position of the lower lumbar spine in the standing posture.

The fourth point, the greater trochanter, is difficult to compare bilaterally because of its size (Fig. 5–8). Therefore, it should be used to

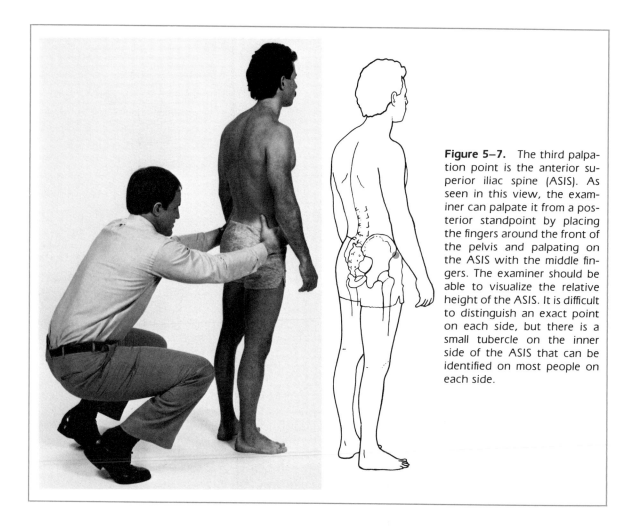

Figure 5–7. The third palpation point is the anterior superior iliac spine (ASIS). As seen in this view, the examiner can palpate it from a posterior standpoint by placing the fingers around the front of the pelvis and palpating on the ASIS with the middle fingers. The examiner should be able to visualize the relative height of the ASIS. It is difficult to distinguish an exact point on each side, but there is a small tubercle on the inner side of the ASIS that can be identified on most people on each side.

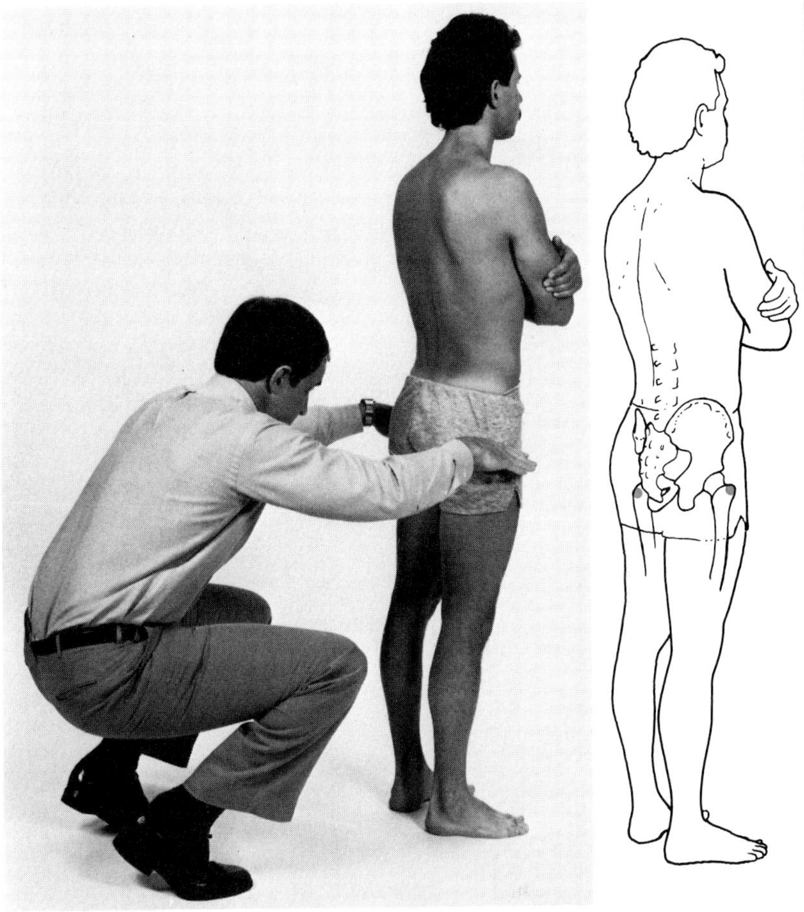

Figure 5–8. The last palpation points in the standing examination are the greater trochanters. It is difficult to distinguish an exact point on either side because of the extensive amount of connective tissue on top of this bony landmark. For this reason it is the least important point in palpation but is used just to add to the information that is found with the previous three palpation points in standing.

help verify frontal plane asymmetries. For example, if the right iliac crest, PSIS, and ASIS are higher when compared with the left, then the greater trochanter should be palpated. If the trochanter is also high on the right and the patient is bearing weight equally on both lower extremities, then the patient has either a skeletally short left lower extremity, an angle difference at the hip, a size variation of one of the ilia, or soft-tissue asymmetries. For the purpose of this text, we prefer to call this type of difference a *frontal plane asymmetry*. Whatever the reason for the asymmetry, the sacral base is now tilted to the left because of the position of the pelvis in the frontal plane. This re-

sults in a compensatory lumbar side bending to the right.[7]

Right side bending results in asymmetrical weight-bearing and increased loading patterns of the lumbopelvic tissues.[7,9,10,19,34] If a frontal plane asymmetry has been determined, small blocks of known thickness can be placed under the foot on the short side (Fig. 5–9).[3] All points can be palpated again in order to assess symmetry.

After placing blocks of the desired thickness under the short side, the patient is asked to equally distribute his weight. The blocks are then removed, and the patient is again asked to equalize his weight. This is repeated several

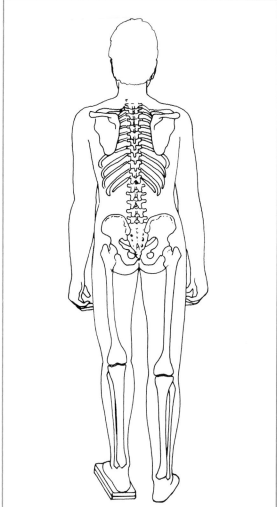

Figure 5–9. Posterior view of the patient in standing examination showing two ⅛'' calibrated blocks under the left foot that balance all four points. These blocks can be taken out and measured as to the difference in the standing examination between the right and left sides.

to change the loading pattern of his lumbopelvic tissues as an initial step in his treatment regimen.

There are other methods of assessing whether one leg is shorter than the other. Most of these tests are conducted in the supine, non-weight-bearing position. However, a person's standing, antigravity mechanics are very different from his body mechanics when he is supine. Therefore, the standing assessment yields more clinically relevant information because it is in the upright postures that a person usually is symptomatic. In the clinic a situp maneuver is often used to measure the functional leg length discrepancy. In this test the patient is asked to sit up from the supine position in order to assess which leg moves farther. If one leg moves forward farther than the other, the interpretation is most often a functional leg length discrepancy owing to a pelvic dysfunction. The interpretation of these findings disregards the neuromuscular control of the movement.

In conducting this situp test the clinician assumes that perfectly symmetrical concentric and eccentric contractions occur on the right and left sides of the trunk and lower extremities. This is an unreasonable assumption because a person who is experiencing pain will guard the injured area and alter muscle activity accordingly. This causes the lumbopelvic segments to move asymmetrically. Therefore, caution must be taken in interpreting the findings of this test as having the same meaning as the antigravity standing evaluation. If we are concerned about the effect of asymmetrical forces reaching tissues, then we need to closely assess the postures and movement patterns that allow this to occur. Drawing conclusions about structural differences from the prone or supine position does not yield functional information because superincumbent and ground forces are removed.

Another finding at the pelvis might be a high iliac crest and ASIS and a low PSIS on the right side. Assuming symmetrical weight-bearing, this could be interpreted as a sagittal plane asymmetry when comparing the right side of the pelvis with the left. In this example the findings appear to indicate that either the right ilium is fixed in a posteriorly rotated position

times. The patient is then asked about his perception of discomfort both while he was on the blocks and while he was off the blocks. If the patient responds that while he was on the blocks the "pressure" decreased or he was more comfortable, then the patient is conveying to the clinician the importance of the need

or the left ilium is fixed in an anterior position. This narrow interpretation ignores the muscle activity of the region resulting from afferent input. That the ilium can become fixed in a posterior or anterior position without significant musculature reaction is questionable. With the current understanding of the anatomy, function, and aging sequence of the sacroiliac joint (Chapter 4), we question whether this joint, especially in men, can become fixed and blocked in one of these positions unless there is significant trauma. This finding may be more representative of an asymmetrical neuromuscular control mechanism than a fixation of bony elements, especially since the afferent-efferent balance of neurologic activity is altered as a result of injury.

Colachis and colleagues[5] used pins placed in the pelvic bones to determine movement. Their conclusions noted that there is a small amount of movement present, with the greatest amount occurring in the position of forward bending from the standing position. Weisl[32] reported movement at 5.6 mm, while Sashin[23] reported an average range of 4 degrees of movement between the sacrum and ilium. The sacroiliac joint also has highly incongruous surfaces and a massive ligamentous support system that also precludes large ranges of motion. Age-related changes and sacroiliac mechanics probably preclude the bones' moving out of place and "getting stuck." Perhaps this is possible in multiparous women or in young people with viscoelastic qualities of their connective tissues that permit hypermobility of joints, but this population is certainly not the majority of mechanical low back pain patients. We are probably dealing with the application of forces that overload the support tissues, rather than with actual movements that are giving rise to the painful stimulus.

Gross Movement Testing

Gross movement testing with the patient in the standing position is vitally important in assessing the response of the various tissues to tensile, compressive, torsional, and shear forces. It is important that the clinician be able to visualize how these forces reach the tissues of the lumbopelvic region in order to interpret the patient's response to these movements. Important information is gleaned because the person's musculoskeletal tissues are moved during weight-bearing. Key questions to ask during the movement testing include whether the movement pattern is making the pain worse and whether it is reproducing the familiar pain, that is, representative of the chief complaint. The standing position is the most important position when evaluating mechanical pain, since the patient has pain during weight-bearing and experiences relief, for the most part, when recumbent. Therefore, the familiar pain must be reproduced in this position in order to proceed with the examination. The supine and prone portions of the assessment are designed to cross check the mechanics of the standing examination.

Gross movement testing includes active forward bending, backward bending, side bending, and any combination of these that alters the manner in which the lumbopelvic tissues bear weight. Overpressure can be applied to any of these movements much in the same manner as when evaluating the extremities (Fig. 5–10).

Forward bending is assessed by watching the complete spine and then the pelvis move in a smooth synchronous manner. The examiner is assessing lumbopelvic rhythm as the forces of forward bending proceed from the cervical spine down into the pelvis.[3] The L4-L5 and L5-S1 segments combine for approximately 45 degrees of motion in this plane, and the clinician should be able to detect whether the lumbar and pelvic regions are moving normally.[33] Visualizing the synchronized movements of the spinal segments as the motion reaches the pelvis and continues around the femurs is more important than simply assessing whether or not the patient can touch the floor. It is important to note if the patient is not moving in a particular region of the spine. This may be the result of either true tightness or protective muscle guarding.

The clinician should apply overpressure to the forward and side bending motions or combinations thereof if this can be done without further injury. In order for overpressure to be correctly applied in forward bending, side bending, or a combination of the two motions, it is important that the pelvis be stabilized. Figure 5–10 shows hand placement over the sacrum to stabilize the sacral base while the overpressure force is applied.

The patient is then asked to backward bend. The clinician again observes the preferred movement pattern. Many patients backward bend by simply hyperextending at the hips. By doing this they avoid increasing the forces that accompany extension of the lumbopelvic region. Figure 5–11 shows how the clinician can control the extension motion, directing the force through the lumbopelvic region by applying a compressive force with the hands through the patient's shoulders. This force is

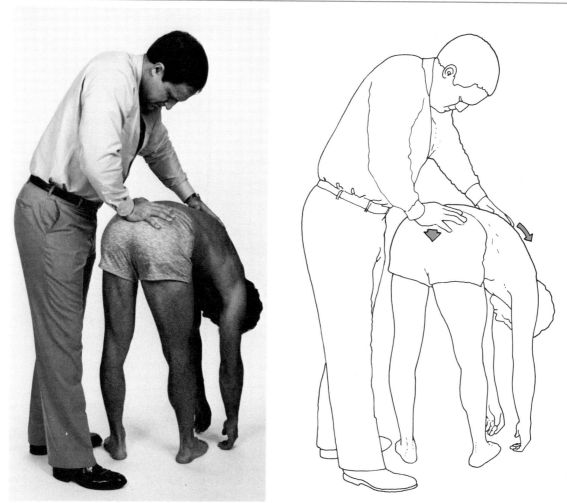

Figure 5–10. Overpressure in forward bending. Note how the examiner's hands are pushing in opposite directions. The reader should visualize the tissues from the skin to the central core as they elongate posterior to the center of rotation and compress anterior to the center of rotation with this maneuver.

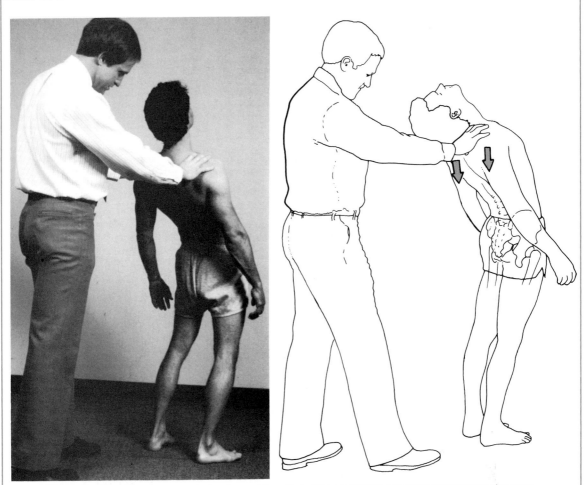

Figure 5–11. Overpressure in backward bending. The examiner can manually retract the scapulae, which focuses the force in the upper part of the lumbar spine, and then a compressive force down into the spine compresses the lumbar vertebrae. Again, the examiner should be able to visualize the lumbopelvic tissues as this force passes through the lumbopelvic region.

applied with an intensity sufficient to create a small, controlled increase in lumbar lordosis or extension.

To assess the movement of backward bending and side bending to the right (Fig. 5–12), the clinician guides the motion with his right hand, first backward and then side bending right. The left hand maintains the compressive force over the top of the left shoulder. This force directs the weight line (compression line)

over the lower lumbar and lumbosacral zygapophysial joints, the sacroiliac joint, and the related tissues on the right side. The left hand gradually increases the compressive force to this area.

This line of compressive force starts at the left shoulder and travels through the midthoracic spine into the contralateral lower lumbar vertebral segments. The line of force travels into the lumbosacral triangle and then reaches the superior aspect of the sacroiliac joint. By this time the right L5-S1 zygapophysial joint has been placed in a closed-pack position, and the force continues through the structures of the sacroiliac joint.

Other combinations of forward bending, backward bending, side bending, and rotation can be used in the same manner to identify the pattern that best reproduces the symptom (Figs. 5–13 and 5–14). Note how the femoral extension in Figure 5–14 enhances the extension moment on the left lumbosacral region. Once the examiner can visualize the direction and result of any force generated into this region, he will be better able to assess the status of the neuromuscular and musculoskeletal systems.

This type of gradual, guided overpressure

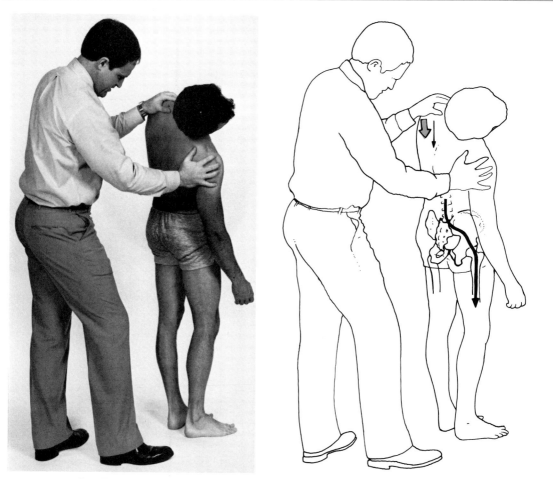

Figure 5–12. Overpressure in backward bending and side bending right. The examiner guides with the right hand and causes a compressive force through the left hand. The examiner should be able to visualize the vertical force from the left hand as it passes down through the shoulder, into and through the thoracic spine, down into the right lumbosacral triangle, and out through the right leg. All those tissues in the right lumbosacral triangle are specifically compressed as the trunk and ground forces reach this region.

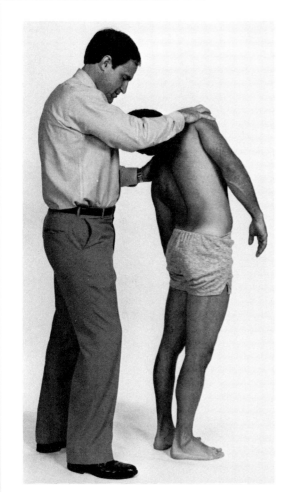

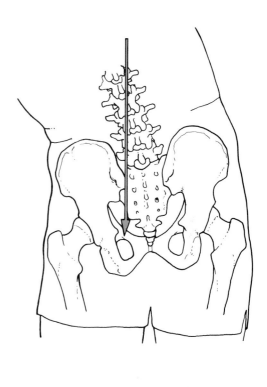

Figure 5–13. Backward bending, side bending to the left, and rotation to the right, with a superior-to-inferior overpressure applied through the right shoulder.

during gross movement testing from the standing position is probably the most important part of the entire assessment because the subsequent supine and prone assessments are designed to substantiate the pain pattern found with gross movement testing. If the clinician cannot reproduce familiar symptoms in gross movement testing, then determining the correct course of the treatment will be difficult.

A comment is necessary regarding the so-called specific mobility testing of the sacroiliac joint. This test and variations of it were origi-

nally designed to evaluate movement of the ilium on the sacrum when the standing person flexes the thigh and hip. As the hip is flexed, the ipsilateral innominate bone moves through an arc best described as posterior torsion. The clinician palpates the PSIS or the ischial tuberosity and follows these bony landmarks moving in an inferior or a downward direction (Fig. 5–15). This motion can be detected if compared with the relatively stationary position of the opposite PSIS or the second sacral spinous process. If a downward motion occurs, sacroiliac

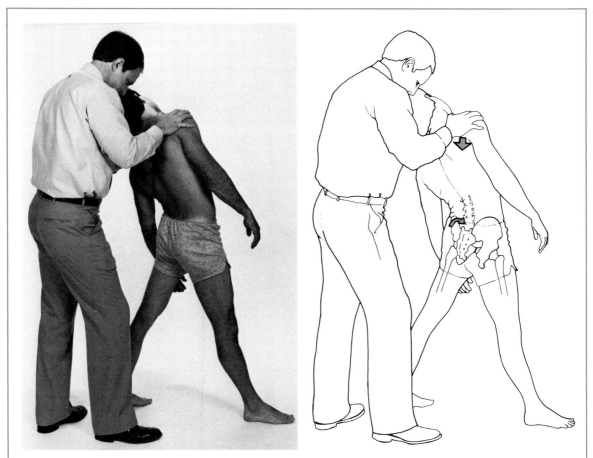

Figure 5–14. Adaptation of the standing examination that increases the extension force in the left lumbosacral triangle by extending the leg. With femoral extension and then backward bending and side bending to the left with overpressure through the right hand, the end-range of extension and compression can be evaluated in the left lumbosacral triangle. The examiner can vary the leg position, trunk position, and overpressure position of the force in any of these examples.

joint movement is considered normal. On the other hand, dysfunction is thought to be present—in particular, a "blocked joint"—if the PSIS or ischial tuberosity moved in an upward direction while the hip was flexing. This interpretation is too restrictive, and does not take into account all of the relevant neuromuscular activity that necessarily occurs with the test.

When a person flexes the right hip while standing, the left hip abductors must be strong enough to stabilize the pelvis in the frontal plane. Nevertheless, the pelvis drops on the opposite side as soon as the leg is lifted from the ground, much in the same manner as the frontal plane tilt of the pelvis during gait. This tilt causes the PSIS and ischial tuberosity to assume a more inferior position when compared with the opposite side. This downward motion is not due to sagittal plane posterior torsion, but rather to frontal plane tilt.

As the person flexes the hip, and the structures on the posterior aspect of the hip become taut, a posterior torsional force is applied to the sacroiliac joint followed by a flexion force on the lumbar spine. If these forces are potentially painful to any of the supporting structures of the low back, the patient reflexively alters the movement to protect the region. Many muscles are involved in stabilizing and moving the trunk and lower extremities. For this reason a more accurate interpretation of an atypical movement pattern of the pelvis during the hip flexion test, or any other mobility test, should simply be "altered lumbopelvic mechanics" rather than "a blocked segment."

SUPINE TESTING

With the patient in a supine position the examiner can evaluate hip mobility and place various forces through the sacroiliac and lumbar joints. Much of the neurologic evaluation can also be performed in this position (see Chapter 2). Table 5–4 outlines the sequence of the supine testing position.

Hip range of motion is an important assessment for low back problems. The examiner must be certain as to when the passive hip motion assessment begins to place forces to the

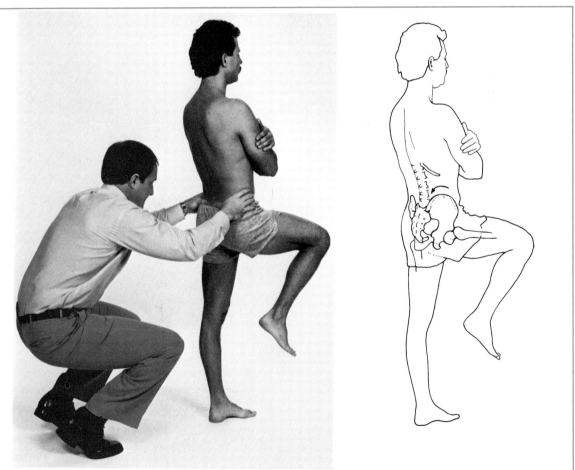

Figure 5–15. The examiner's palpating thumb is at the "shelf" underneath the PSIS, and the patient is asked to actively hip flex. A normal finding would be an inferior motion of the right thumb as the patient actively flexes the right femur.

TABLE 5–4.   Supine Testing: Substantiate Finding of the GMT

A. Progressive flexion (tensile forces utilizing the femur)
1. Passive hip flexion
2. Posterior torsion of the ilium
3. Lumbosacral flexion
4. Lumbar flexion
B. Figure 4 (Faber)
C. Straight-leg raising (SLR)
D. Stresses to the pelvis via femur
E. Neurologic screening (Chapter 2)

pelvis and then the lumbar spine. For example, as the femur is passively flexed, the hip joint capsule unwinds and the hip joint becomes "open" or "loose-packed." As the hip is moved from the neutral position toward full flexion, the hip extensors are stretched and the femur, in essence, becomes part of the innominate (Fig. 5–16). As passive hip flexion continues, the motion places a posterior torsional stress of the ilium on the sacrum. There is then a small posterior rotary accommodation of the ilium on the sacrum at the sacroiliac joint.

Once the limits of the sacroiliac joint accommodation are reached and all of the tissue slack is taken up, the ilium and sacrum move as a unit. The continued force of passive hip flexion results in lumbosacral flexion. This inferior migration of the superior articulating process of S1 on the inferior articulating process of the L5 vertebra results in a flexion force at the L5-S1 segment. This motion continues to involve the remainder of the lumbar vertebrae as the tissues tighten in flexion from below upward. Therefore, it is important that the examiner know how far up the kinetic chain movement occurs.

Other hip motions are assessed, and care is taken to determine what is actually hip motion versus pelvic and lumbar motions. The Figure 4 test, or Faber position, is an excellent method to use to assess the range of motion of the hip joint (Fig. 5–17). Asymmetrical differences in the motion between the right and left sides may be revealed. This is especially important to note in patients with unilateral low back pain.

The Figure 4 position moves the intertro-

chanteric line of the femur away from the ilium and the pubis. This has the effect of placing a tensile force on a significant portion of the hip joint capsule, especially the iliofemoral and pubofemoral portions of the reinforcing capsular ligament (Fig. 5–18). For this reason it is an excellent assessment of the flexibility of the hip joint capsule. If the hip adductor muscles are thought to be the cause of the limited range of motion in the Figure 4 position, a contract-relax technique to the adductors can help to distinguish between muscle tightness and connective tissue shortening of the capsule.

A tight hip joint capsule can contribute to excessive forces that reach the lumbopelvic joints.[18,27,28] Consider the person who walks a great deal at work. Each step the person takes requires her or him to create a hyperextension moment at the hip for effective pushoff. If the person has a tight hip joint capsule, the lower extremity is not placed behind the body by femoral extension, but rather by anterior torsion and rotation of the pelvis and eventual extension of the lumbar spine. The attempt to extend the hip tightens the anterior hip capsular tissues and causes excessive anterior torsion of the ilium on the sacrum, a forward and downward movement of the sacrum, resulting in increased lumbosacral extension and hyperextension of the lumbar spine. Any of these tissues may be symptomatic, and unless the hip range of motion is restored, an abnormal stress reaches the lumbopelvic tissues, contributing to continued damage and prolonged symptoms.

A positive Figure 4 sign may be an indication that femoral extension is limited. If the person with a positive Figure 4 attempts to maintain the same stride length during gait, increased extension stresses to the lumbar spine result. If a limitation in the Figure 4 in the supine position is confirmed, and backward bending and side bending to that side increase familiar symptoms in the standing examination, then this represents a *match*. A *match* is defined as reproduction of the familiar pain described by the patient with a similar combination of stresses in a different position during the evaluation process.

In the previous example the *match* represents backward bending and side bending to

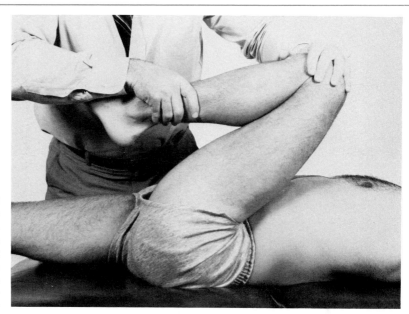

Figure 5–16. Supine lying examination, passive hip flexion. The examiner should visualize the hip as it unwinds and comes into an open-pack position at 90 degrees of hip flexion, and then the transmission of forces to the extensor of the hip, causing a posterior rotary moment on the ilium and ending in spinal flexion. This is another example of directing forces into and through the lumbopelvic region during the examination process for the purpose of provoking the familiar pain.

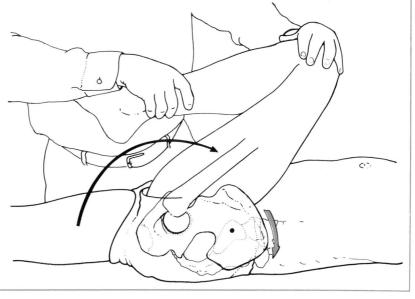

the right (BBSB-R), increasing familiar pain and a positive Figure 4 (decreased femoral extension) on the right. It is common to find a tight hip structure on the side of the low back pain.[27]

The supine lying evaluation continues by performing the straight-leg raise test. The maneuver places a tensile stress to the sciatic nerve and its nerve roots. A positive finding represents reproduction of familiar leg pain as the leg is elevated.[24] If the clinician recognizes this finding, then he or she should maintain the position and observe the changes in the perception of pain. If the pain peripheralizes or

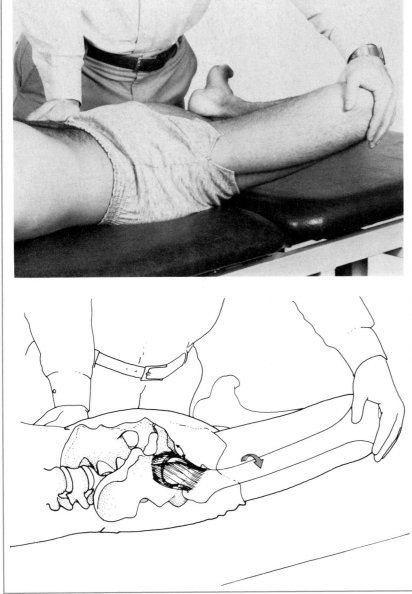

Figure 5–17. Figure 4 or Faber position, which shows passive flexion, abduction, and external rotation. The examiner should be able to visualize the passive stretching of the anterior hip muscles from an anterior to a posterior aspect through and into the hip joint capsule. This stretch is mainly to the iliofemoral ligament, which travels inferiorly and laterally from the rim of the acetabulum to the inner trochanteric line.

moves distal, this adds to the significance of the test. This finding represents possible irritation of the nerve root complex.

The straight-leg raise test can be augmented by combining hip flexion with slight femoral adduction and internal rotation. This position places maximal stretch on the sciatic nerve and the L4-S2 nerve roots, owing to the course of the sciatic nerve as it proceeds lateral to the ischial tuberosity (Fig. 5–19). The conclusions of this test should be combined with other positive findings of the assessment so that a judg-

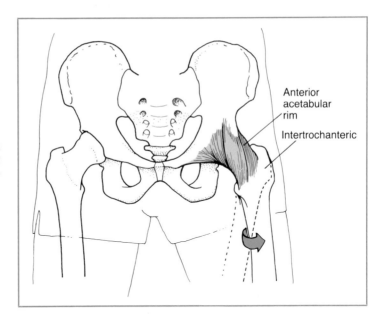

Figure 5–18. Hip capsular mechanics showing a stretch of the iliofemoral and pubofemoral ligaments with the Figure 4 position.

ment can be made as to the mechanics of the painful low back syndrome.

From the supine position a variety of stresses can be placed to the sacroiliac joints and surrounding structures. Figure 5–20 shows the long axis of the femur placed in approximately the same plane as the sacroiliac joint. From this position a graded force is applied through the long axis of the femur to create a shear force at the sacroiliac joint. This force is di-

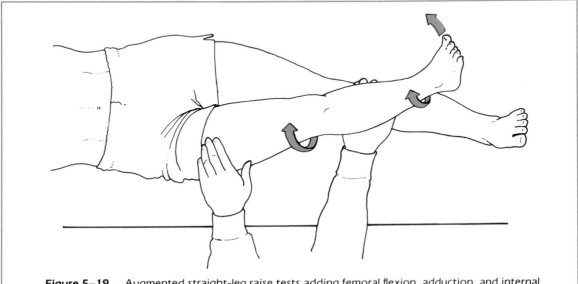

Figure 5–19. Augmented straight-leg raise tests adding femoral flexion, adduction, and internal rotation. This change in mechanics increases the tensile force on the sciatic nerve as a result of the nerve's lateral relation to the ischial tuberosity.

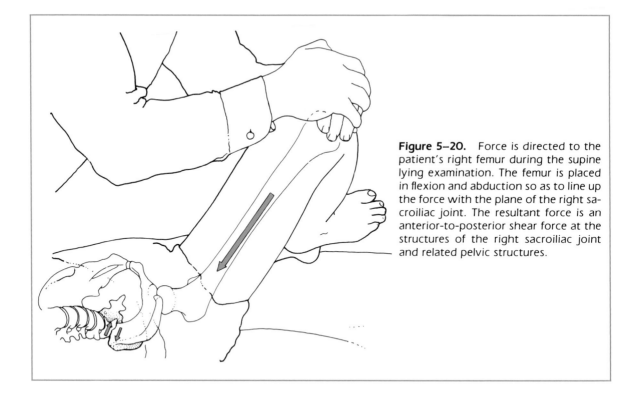

Figure 5–20. Force is directed to the patient's right femur during the supine lying examination. The femur is placed in flexion and abduction so as to line up the force with the plane of the right sacroiliac joint. The resultant force is an anterior-to-posterior shear force at the structures of the right sacroiliac joint and related pelvic structures.

rected on a line through the patella and into the femur. The force then travels through the length of the femur to reach the hip joint. Here, the superior and posterior aspects of the femoral head articulate with the posterior acetabulum. The articular cartilages become compressed. The force continues into the pelvis and creates an anterior-to-posterior shear at the sacroiliac joint. Once this small tissue deformation has taken place, the force then travels through the soft tissues of the buttock and into the table.

If this maneuver provokes familiar pain, then the clinician can deduce that any or all of the tissues could be involved in the pain syndrome. If this test is positive on one side, and the patient has unilateral pain at the sacroiliac region, and the standing extension and side bending test is painful to that side, then this represents a series of *matches.*

Using the femur as a lever, a variety of stresses can be directed to the musculoskeletal structures of the lumbopelvic region. Figures 5–21 and 5–22 show some of the stresses to this region. The position of the femur and the amount and direction of the stresses applied help to identify the area involved in the painful syndrome. The clinician must be cognizant of how and when the stresses progressively reach the pelvis and are transferred into the lumbar tissues. If the pelvic or lumbar structures are involved in the painful syndrome, the patient should respond with a complaint of familiar pain each time the examiner directs similar stresses to the region, whether from a standing, supine, or prone lying position.

PRONE TESTING

The patient is asked to lie prone. Table 5–5 outlines the sequence of the prone lying examination. A pillow can be placed under the abdomen to support a neutral position of the lumbar spine. The clinician should consis-

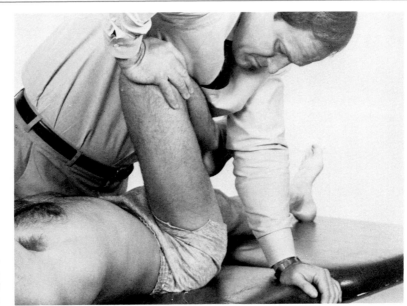

Figure 5–21. Posterior-to-anterior force directed to the femur in a flexed and vertical position. The resultant force is a compression at the anterior aspect of the sacroiliac joint and a slight gap at the posterior aspect of the sacroiliac joint. It is a direct posterior-to-anterior force at the pelvis.

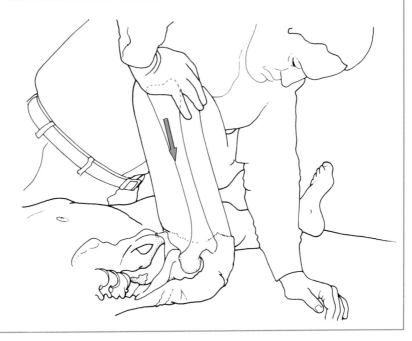

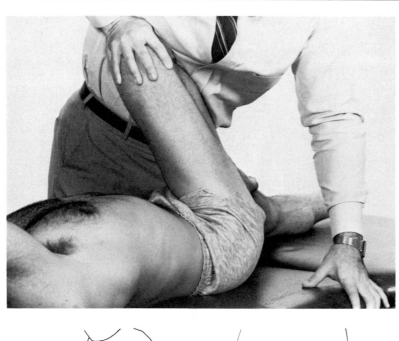

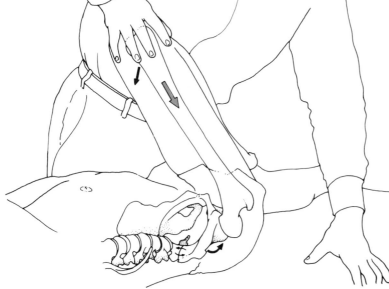

Figure 5–22. Force generated through the femur into the pelvis with the femur in flexion and adduction. The examiner should place a long axis force down through the femur until all of the tissues have become taut, and then a small adduction force is imparted to the femur, which causes an extreme compression at the anterior aspect of the sacroiliac joint and a significant gapping stress at the posterior aspect. If the long axis force is not generated through the femur to the pelvis in the initial parts of this testing, then a significant compression force to the anterior labrum and iliopectineal bursa results, and the patient experiences pain in the pubis. This is just another example of a force that can be imparted to the right pelvic structures to determine if it causes pain.

TABLE 5–5.   Prone Testing: Substantiate Finding of the GMT

A. Knee flexion
B. Progressive extension (compressive forces utilizing femur)
    1. Hip extension
    2. Anterior torsion of the ilium
    3. Lumbosacral extension
    4. Lumbar extension
C. P-A stresses to sacrum/ilium
D. P-A stresses to lumbar spine
E. Palpation
F. Neurologic screening (Chapter 2)

tently use the same method of prone positioning with each patient. This helps to standardize as much of the examination as possible in order to decrease the variability of findings among patients.

The rectus femoris muscle is first assessed by passively flexing the knee (Fig. 5–23). This muscle attaches to the superior aspect of the acetabulum and the anterior inferior iliac spine. The examiner pays attention to and palpates any movement of the pelvis as the knee is passively flexed. If there is a decrease in the length or an increase in the stiffness of the rectus femoris muscle, then flexion of the knee can cause an anterior torsional stress to the ilium because of its anterior attachments to the pelvis.[4,13] This stress can then be translated up into the lumbar spine as backward bending or lumbar extension.

The examiner proceeds by internally and externally rotating the hip (Fig. 5–24). This repeats a portion of the hip motion assessment from the supine test and provides another piece of information regarding the mobility of the hip joint. Unlike in the supine test, the hip joint is in a relatively close-packed position. These findings should closely correlate with the results of the Figure 4 test. Asymmetrical tightness in the hip joint, especially on the painful side, plays a major role in the force transmission to and through the lumbopelvic region.

After examination of the hip the clinician begins to assess the pelvis. The clinician must visualize the approximate plane of the sacroiliac joint, taking into consideration that the sacrum is wider anteriorly and superiorly than

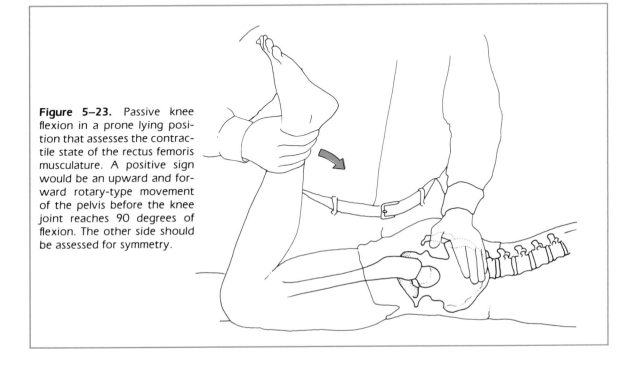

Figure 5–23. Passive knee flexion in a prone lying position that assesses the contractile state of the rectus femoris musculature. A positive sign would be an upward and forward rotary-type movement of the pelvis before the knee joint reaches 90 degrees of flexion. The other side should be assessed for symmetry.

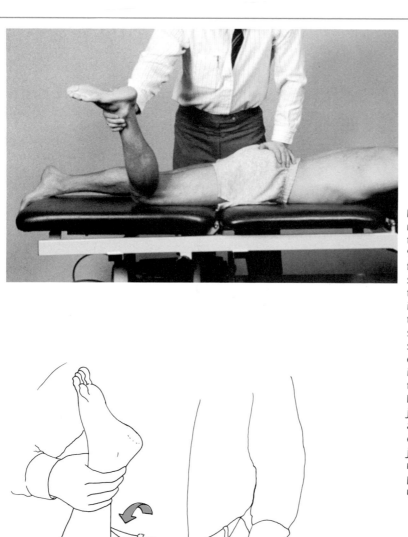

Figure 5–24. Passive internal and external rotation of the hip joint with the knee at 90 degrees of flexion. The findings of this evaluation should be similar to Figure 4 in the supine lying position; that is, tightness in external rotation in supine should also be seen in prone. The examiner should note the change in capsular position with the hip in flexion (supine lying) and the hip in extension (prone lying). In prone lying the hip joint is more close-packed, and one should notice an increased tightness if the hip joint capsule is tight. This almost always matches the supine lying examination in Figure 4.

posteriorly and inferiorly. If the clinician is unaware of the joint plane and the depth of the tissues related to the sacroiliac joint, then the results from application of forces will be difficult to interpret. Gentle and graded forces are introduced. The clinician should be able to visualize the transference of the shear force through the sacroiliac joint as it passes along the long axis of the femur. Where in the progression the patient responds to familiar pain represents the depth or level of the injured tissue.

Many techniques are used to apply forces through the pelvis. With the person's knees flexed, the clinician grasps the anterior distal aspect of the femur with one hand and places the other hand over the ipsilateral posterior ilium. The clinician then passively extends and adducts the femur in a graded manner until he palpates motion at the pelvis (Fig. 5–25). The kinesiological analysis of this force is as follows: as the femur is extended and adducted the hip joint becomes close-packed because the capsule and the iliopsoas and other hip flexor muscles become taut. The tightening of these soft tissues results in a rotary stress to the ilium and accommodation by the sacroiliac joint.

As the passive femoral extension continues, the motion of the pelvis and sacrum creates an extension force at the L5-S1 zygapophyseal joint as the superior articulating process of the sacrum moves on the inferior articulating process of the L5 segment. Coupled with this extension moment is an anterior shear force between the sacrum and the L5 segment. It is logical to conclude that this combination of extension and shear results in a tightening of the iliolumbar ligaments bilaterally, an increased compression of the articular surfaces of the L5-S1 zygapophyseal joint, an increased compression to the posterior aspect of the intervertebral disc, and an increased tensile force to the anterior aspect of the disc.

The motion continues further to include the L5-L4, L4-L3, L3-L2 segments, and so on. The protective response of the musculature owing to injury should be recognized. If the forces that accompany the motion generate potentially destructive stimuli to any of the tissues,

the clinician should be able to palpate a protective guarding contraction of the surrounding muscles as the extension force continues. Injury decreases the tissues' threshold to stimuli. A negative finding is painless full range.

The reader should recognize the similarities between this motion and that of the backward bending and side bending standing test. If this motion caused increased pain during the standing examination, the comparable motion in the prone lying examination should elicit a similar response. This represents another example of a *match* that is indicative of a mechanical disorder.

The prone examination continues with the application of compression forces over the posterior aspect of the sacrum. By placing the hand directly over the patient's midsacrum, the examiner applies a posterior-to-anterior shear force to the sacroiliac joint (Fig. 5–26). This stresses the supporting structures of the sacroiliac joint and compresses the intervening soft tissues under the examiner's hands. The object of this test is not to quantify mobility, but rather to apply a force that may reproduce the patient's pain.

The examiner's hand can then be placed on the PSIS of the ilium (Fig. 5–27). A stress is applied along the plane of the sacroiliac joint, resulting in an anterior rotary moment to the ilium. Reproduction of familiar pain is a positive finding.

Another test involves the examiner's placing his thumb on the skin over the sacrum parallel to the sacroiliac joint line (Fig. 5–28). The thumb is placed just medial to the PSIS. The examiner's other hand is placed over the thumb and a gradual posterior-to-anterior force is applied by the hand through the thumb and into the tissues (Fig. 5–29). This posterior-to-anterior force compresses the skin, fat, thoracolumbar fascia, erector spinae aponeurosis, and multifidus muscle. It then reaches the lateral border of the sacrum, which results in a shear force of the sacrum on the ilium.

These tests, like most sacroiliac joint tests, attempt to place controlled forces through the tissues. If symptoms cannot be reproduced and the forces have been specifically directed to the sacroiliac joint structures, the pain is prob-

Text continued on page 158

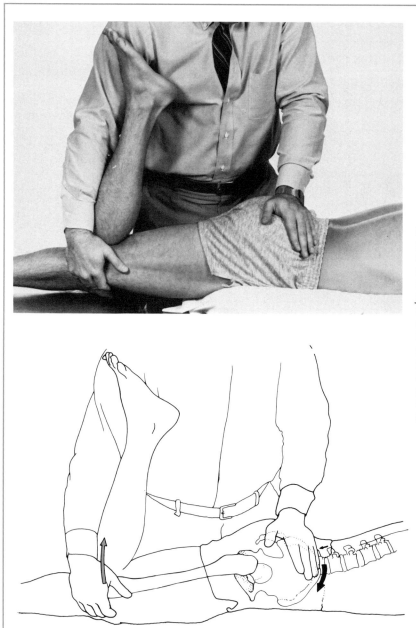

Figure 5–25. Prone lying passive femoral extension. The examiner should visualize the anterior femoral musculature becoming taut, and the hip joint capsule becoming taut, which then imparts an anterior rotary moment to the ilium and eventually a flexion moment to the sacrum, which is an extension force to the lumbosacral junction. Completed motion causes an extension up through the lumbar spine.

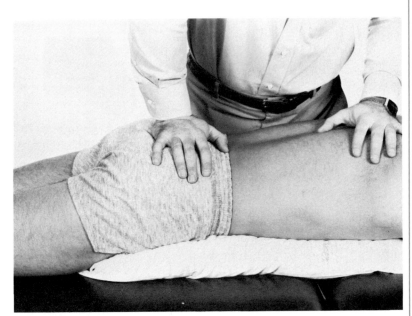

Figure 5–26. Posterior-to-anterior force is directed through the skin into the mid-aspect of the sacrum, causing a direct posterior-to-anterior shear of the sacrum on the ilium. The examiner should not quantify motion, but rather gradually introduce this force into the sacrum, which stresses those structures that support the sacrum as it is suspended between the ilia.

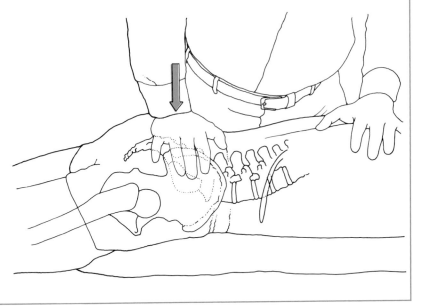

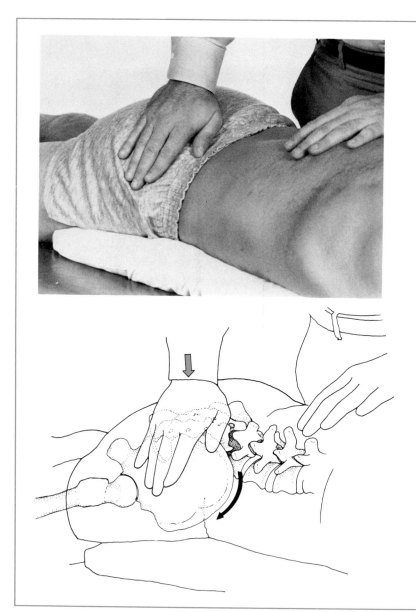

Figure 5–27. Prone lying examination. Posterior-to-anterior rotary force imparted to the posterior superior iliac spine and the right ilium. Gradual progression of force stresses those tissues that stabilize the right side of the pelvis.

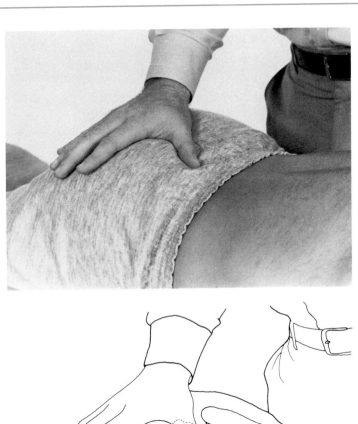

Figure 5–28. The examiner places the thenar eminence of the thumb at the sacral apex and rotates the thumb to bump into the right PSIS. This places the thumb along the sacrum. The thumb is placed in this position so that force can be directed through it into the posterior musculature of the dorsal sacrum and then along the sacroiliac joint, creating a posterior-to-anterior shear.

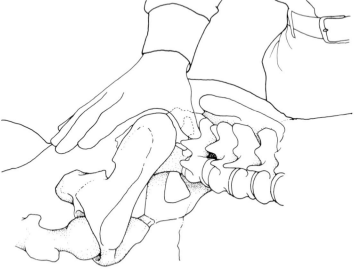

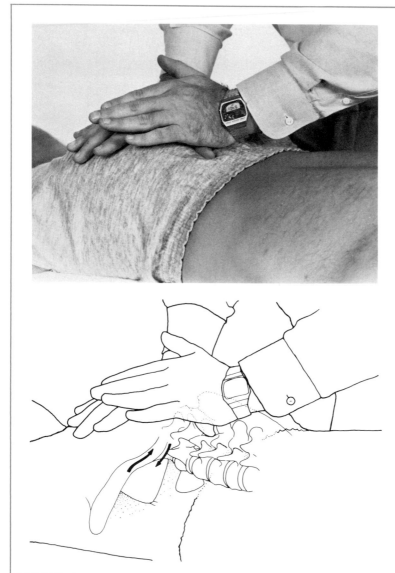

Figure 5–29. By using the other hand over top of the thumb positioned along the sacrum, the examiner can direct the force posterior to anterior until all the slack is taken out of the tissue. Then an angular force downward and outward can be placed, simulating shear force from a posterior-to-anterior aspect of the sacrum on the ilium along the sacroiliac joint. The examiner should visualize the stress being placed at this region, as the sacrum is wider anteriorly than posteriorly. This mainly stresses the strong ligamentous structure of the sacroiliac joint region, both anteriorly and posteriorly.

ably *not* due to mechanical dysfunction of the sacroiliac joint.

The prone lying examination continues with the assessment of the lumbar spine. The examiner begins by placing the hypothenar aspect of the hand on the skin of the superior dorsal aspect of the sacrum and applying a posterior-to-anterior force (Fig. 5–30). This results in an extension force on the lumbosacral junction. The extension force is thus created by

pressure over the central aspect of the sacrum, rather than by the previously described long-lever technique using the femur.

The remaining lumbar spine segments are tested in the same manner. The examiner places his hand on the skin and presses to impact on the spinous process. A posterior-to-anterior force is applied to each segment (Fig. 5–31). As the force progresses into the spinous process it travels down the bony column into

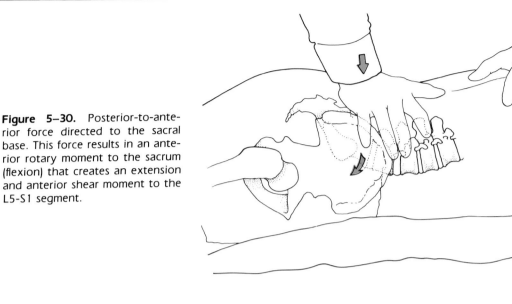

Figure 5–30. Posterior-to-anterior force directed to the sacral base. This force results in an anterior rotary moment to the sacrum (flexion) that creates an extension and anterior shear moment to the L5-S1 segment.

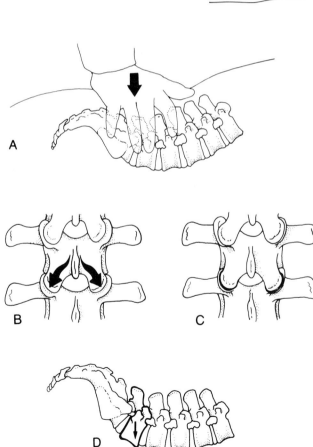

A

B

C

D

Figure 5–31. Four-step progression showing the force transmitted from the examiner's hand to the spinous process and through the lumbar spine into the abdominal cavity: A, Purchasing on the spinous process; B, force transmitted through the spinous process down to the lamina into the inferior articulating process; C, continuing progression down through the spinous process into the lamina, squeezing the apophyseal joints together and causing a small extension force of the inferior articulating process, sliding down the superior articulating process; and D, the final aspect of the of the force generated through this system is a small posterior-to-anterior shear at the bone-disc-bone interface. The force is then generated from the lumbar spine into the abdominal contents. This is just another example of analyzing the force production from the examiner into the patient through any test in the evaluation process. If this increases the familiar pain, an analysis of vectors and forces should be carried out to substantiate or match the standing examination.

the lamina bilaterally and into the inferior articulating process (IAP) of the vertebra above. As the posterior-to-anterior force gently proceeds, the IAP articular cartilage is engaged into the articular cartilage of the superior articulating process (SAP) of the vertebra immediately caudal. The force causes these two surfaces to compress. Because of the lordotic position of these two vertebrae, an extension moment is generated.

The force is subsequently transferred to the subchondral bone plate of the articular processes, the bony trabecular system of the vertebral pedicle and body, and finally to the intervertebral disc. This posterior-to-anterior force that began at the spinous process ends with a posterior-to-anterior shear to the vertebral body–intervertebral disc interface of the vertebral segment above the tested level. The goal is not to quantify the amount of motion or diagnose the specific tissue, but to assess the capability of the tissues to tolerate these stresses. This is carried out on the remaining lumbar vertebral segments.

Other extension stresses can be applied to the lumbar spine in different ways. For example, while remaining in a prone position, the patient is asked to prop himself up on his elbows. This position represents end-range extension of the lumbar spine. The examiner then applies a posterior-to-anterior force (Fig. 5–32). A positive finding would be pain with the introduction of the stress.

To complete the assessement of the tolerance of the lumbar spine to passive motion, the examiner can introduce a rotary force in much the same manner. The examiner places his hand at the midlumbar region opposite the painful side lateral to the spinous processes and introduces a posterior-to-anterior force to the skin, progressing into the fatty layer, fascia, aponeurosis of the superficial erector spinae, and deep erector spinae and finally onto the transverse process and the lateral aspect of the vertebrae. Once the tissue has been compressed between the examiner's hand and the lateral vertebrae, the force is continued to produce a rotary force.

For example, if a stress was applied to the right side, the resultant force would be rotation to the left. The motion creates an engagement of the inferior articulating process on the superior articulating process and a rotary and shear force at the intervertebral disc (see Chapter 4, Fig. 4–10). This stress can be applied lateral to the spinous processes between the iliac crest and the 12th rib. The key is to reproduce the symptom and at the same time evaluate the migration of the applied force.

If the examiner is able to successfully reproduce the symptom in this position, he or she can reposition the patient to further assess the mechanics. For example, if the patient had pain on the right with passive femoral extension at the middle range of motion, pain with central force directed to the spinous process at the lower lumbar segments, and pain with a left rotary force at the same level, then the examiner can reposition the patient to confirm these painful mechanics. When the patient rises on his elbows, the lumbar spine is placed in extension. Now an applied posterior-to-anterior vertical force will probably elicit the painful response more quickly. The examiner has thus confirmed the painful force, causing a nociceptive response, and can use this important information in biomechanically counseling the patient during the treatment process.

Palpation

The last portion of the prone examination is palpation. The back can be palpated in a number of ways. As with other aspects of the assessment system, we suggest that the examiner palpate this and any other musculoskeletal area with a sequence that is comfortable and follows a logical progression. The palpation examination attempts to identify any painful areas in the soft tissues, tenderness, spasm, and defects, dissimilarities in size, or inconsistencies of the musculature, subcutaneous tissues, and skin.

The unaffected region is palpated first. This can be done by first outlining the borders of the last rib, the iliac crest, and the spinous processes. Lateral to the erector spinae muscle is

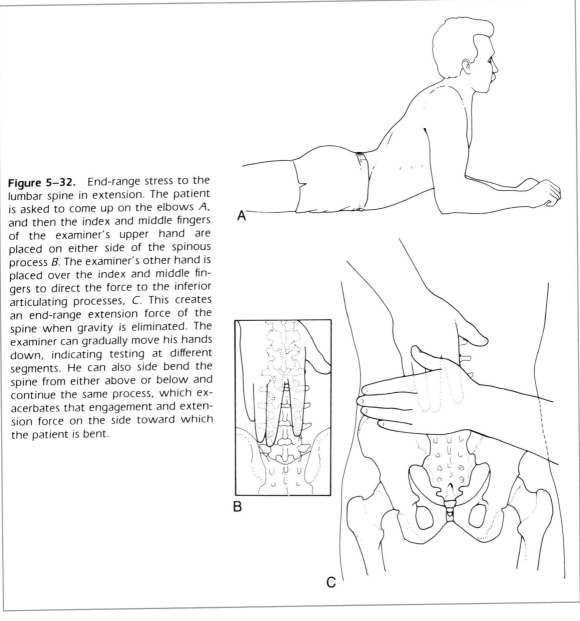

Figure 5–32. End-range stress to the lumbar spine in extension. The patient is asked to come up on the elbows *A*, and then the index and middle fingers of the examiner's upper hand are placed on either side of the spinous process *B*. The examiner's other hand is placed over the index and middle fingers to direct the force to the inferior articulating processes, *C*. This creates an end-range extension force of the spine when gravity is eliminated. The examiner can gradually move his hands down, indicating testing at different segments. He can also side bend the spine from either above or below and continue the same process, which exacerbates that engagement and extension force on the side toward which the patient is bent.

the posterior extent of the external oblique. This area has a softer, spongier consistency than the more medial erector spinae tissues. As the palpating fingers move medial from the external oblique muscle, the lateral border of the erector spinae is located. The soft tissue can be palpated from the iliac crest to the last rib. The examiner is looking for any painful or soft-tis-sue changes that may signify injury or protective muscle spasm.

The lateral aspect of the erector spinae muscle is the anatomical location of the lateral raphe (Chapter 3). At the inferior aspect of this raphe, at the level of the iliac crest, is an important connective tissue juncture (see Fig. 3–11). This is where the thoracolumbar fascia, the lateral aspect of the iliocostalis lumborum tendon, the attachments of the deep erector spinae muscle, the quadratus lumborum muscle, and the lateral one third of the iliolumbar ligament converge to attach to the iliac crest. The cluneal nerves also pass over the iliac crest and near this juncture (see Fig. 2–13). This anatomical region is frequently tender to palpation, especially in the patient with bending and lifting injuries.

Consider the forces that this site must withstand with a forward bending and side bending movement. Because the axis for flexion of the lumbar spine is located in the intervertebral disc, the tissues at this attachment are located a significant distance from this axis.[33] The lumbar tissues must, therefore, tolerate considerable stress as a person bends forward. The examiner should identify this region to determine if these tissues might be injured and, more important, correlate this with the history and the standing, supine, and prone evaluation.

For example, if a patient with a lifting injury presents with symptoms that can be reproduced with forward bending and side bending to the right in standing, and lumbar flexion created by the end-range hip flexion test in supine is also painful, and if palpation to this region is quite tender, then it is reasonable to conclude that tensile forces are responsible for the painful syndrome. These findings represent a *match*.

The examiner can proceed by placing his palpating finger at the thickest portion of the erector spinae and palpating progressively deep into this tissue along a line from the iliac crest to the last rib, visualizing the anatomy during the palpation.

The region of the supraspinous and interspinous ligaments is then palpated to elicit tenderness. This palpation includes the specific regions on each side of the spinous process and the interspinous space. If tenderness elicited by this palpation is the only positive finding, then the examiner has little on which to base a treatment program. However, tenderness from this specific palpation that matches the history and findings from the clinical examination yields useful information, and can be interpreted as indicating injured tissue.

SUMMARY

The key to the lumbopelvic examination is directing controlled forces into lumbar, pelvic, and hip tissues. Each clinical test attempts to apply various degrees of compressive, tensile, shear, or torsional stresses. The shear and rotational movements at each specific intersegmental level of the lumbar spine and sacroiliac region are too small to be meaningfully quantified by the examiner. Therefore, the emphasis of the examination should be on the types of force applied rather than on the quantity of movement.

These stresses can be applied in many positions. The goal is to reproduce familiar pain in the standing examination and then substantiate the nociceptive response by the application of similar forces in the supine and prone positions. Certainly the sitting and sidelying positions can be used if they provide the examiner with meaningful information that also provides a *match* to the findings in the standing examination. Rather than being concerned with the exact tissue of injury, the examiner is attempting to determine the stresses that are responsible for the injury-reinjury process. Recognition of these destructive stresses is the most important aspect on which to base a treatment program.

REFERENCES

1. Andriacchi T, Sabiston P, DeHaven K, et al: Ligament: Injury and repair. In Woo SLY, Buckwalter JA (eds): Injury and Repair of the Musculoskeletal Soft Tissues. Park Ridge, Ill, American Academy of Orthopedic Surgeons, 1988.
2. Bortz WM: The disuse syndrome. West J Med 141:691, 1984.
3. Calliet R: Low Back Pain Syndrome, 2nd ed. Philadelphia, FA Davis, 1981.
4. Carew TJ, Ghez C: Muscles and muscle receptors. In Kandel ER, Schwartz JS (eds): Principles of Neural Science, 2nd ed. New York, Elsevier, 1985, p. 443.
5. Colachis SD, Worden RE, Bechtol CO: Movement of the sacroiliac joint in the adult male: A preliminary report. Arch Phys Med Rehabil 44:490, 1963.
6. Finneson BE: Low Back Pain, 2nd ed. Philadelphia, JB Lippincott, 1980.
7. Friberg O: Clinical symptoms and biomechanics of lumbar spine and hip joint. Spine 6:643, 1983.
8. Fullenlove TM, Williams AJ: Comparative roentgen

findings in symptomatic and asymptomatic backs. JAMA 168:572, 1957.

9. Giles LG, Taylor JR: Lowback pain associated with leg length inequality. Spine 6:510, 1981.

10. Gofton JP: Studies in osteoarthritis of the hip and leg length disparity. Can Med Assoc J 104:791, 1971.

11. Harris RI, MacNab I: Structural changes in the intervertebral discs. J Bone Joint Surg [Br] 36B:304, 1954.

12. Kellett J: Acute soft tissue injuries—a review of the literature. Med Sci Sports Exerc 18:489, 1986.

13. Komi PV: Training of muscle strength and power: Interaction of neuromotoric, hypertrophic and mechanical factors. Int J Sports Med 7(Suppl):10, 1986.

14. Magora A, Schwartz A: Relation between the low back pain syndrome and X-ray findings. Scand J Rehabil Med 8:115, 1976.

15. McPoil TG, Grocato RS: The foot and ankle: biomechanical evaluation and treatment. In Gould JA (ed): Orthopaedic and Sports Physical Therapy, 2nd ed. St. Louis, CV Mosby, 1990.

16. Moufarrij NA, Hardy RW, Weinstein MA: Computed tomographic, myelographic, and operative findings in patients with suspected herniated lumbar discs. Neurosurgery 12:184, 1983.

17. Nachemson A: Work for all, for those with low back pain as well. Clin Orthop 179:77, 1983.

18. Offierski CM, MacNab I: Hip-spine syndrome. Spine 8:316, 1983.

19. Pope MH, Bevins T, Wilder DG, Frymoyer JW: The relationship between anthropometric, postural, muscular, and mobility characteristics of males ages 18-55. Spine 10:644, 1985.

20. Root ML, Orien WP, Weed JH: Clinical biomechanics: Normal and abnormal function of the foot, vol 2. Los Angeles, Clinical Biomechanics Corp., 1977.

21. Rothman RH: A study of computer-assisted tomography. Spine 9:548, 1984.

22. Sandstrom J, Hansson T, Jonson R, et al: The bone mineral content of the lumbar spine in patients with chronic low back pain. Spine 10:158, 1985.

23. Sashin D: A critical analysis of the anatomy and the pathological changes of the SI joints. J Bone Joint Surg [Am] 12:891, 1930.

24. Shiging X, Qanzhi Z, Dehao F: Significance of the straight leg raising test in the diagnosis and clinical evaluation of lower lumbar intervertebral disc protrusion. J Bone Joint Surg [Am] 69A:518, 1987.

25. Splithoff CA: Lumbosacral junction: Roentgenographic comparison of patients with and without backache. JAMA 152:1610, 1953.

26. Stone MH: Implications for connective tissue and bone alterations resulting from resistance exercise training. Med Sci Sports Exerc 20(Suppl):S162, 1988.

27. Thurston AJ: Spinal and pelvic kinematics in osteoarthrosis of the hip joint. Spine 10:467, 1985.

28. Thurston AJ, Whittle MW, Stokes IAF: Spinal and pelvic movement during walking: A method of study. Engin Med 10:219, 1981.

29. Torgeson R, Dotler WE: Comparative roentgenographic study of the symptomatic and asymptomatic lumbar spine. J Bone Joint Surg [Am] 58A:850, 1976.

30. Urban J, Maroudas A: The chemistry of the intervertebral disc in relation to its physiological functions and requirements. Clin Rheum Dis 6:51, 1980.

31. van der Muelen JCH: Present state of knowledge on processes of healing in collagen structures. Int J Sports Med 3:4, 1982.

32. Weisl H: The movements of the sacroiliac joint. Acta Anat (Basel) 23:80, 1955.

33. White AA, Panjabi MM: Clinical Biomechanics of the Spine. Philadelphia, JB Lippincott, 1978.

34. Winter RB, Pinto WC: Pelvic obliquity: Its causes and treatment. Spine 11:225, 1986.

6

TREATMENT OF LUMBOPELVIC DISORDERS

Up to this point, considerable effort has been made to detail the functional anatomy of the lumbopelvic region, and to utilize this information to form an evaluation system appropriate for mechanical low back disorders. This information, coupled with an understanding of exercise science and the basic science of soft-tissue healing, forms the basis for this chapter, which is devoted to the treatment of mechanical low back disorders.

PHILOSOPHY OF TREATMENT

There are three underlying concepts in the philosophical framework for a rehabilitation program:

1. With an understanding of the functional anatomy of the spine, mechanical low back disorders can be treated using much of the same treatment philosophy as that used in the rehabilitation of mechanical disorders of the extremities. By this is meant treatment that encourages early activity at an appropriate point in the healing process, and an emphasis on the restoration of function.

2. No modalities or treatment interventions are currently available that "heal" injured tissue. It is recognized that although the human body has enormous potential for healing, most injured tissue will never be restored to the exact structure and function it had in the preinjured state. Therefore, the role of the clinician is to guide the patient through a healing

process that promotes function as early as possible, and to provide the patient with the opportunity to be better prepared for self-management.

3. Oftentimes it does not matter what tissue is involved, but rather identifying the abnormal or poorly tolerated stresses that converge into the region and stimulate the nociceptive system, giving rise to pain. Treatment is designed to better prepare the patient to avoid, eliminate, or deal with these stresses.

Treatment of the lumbopelvic region is based on an understanding of the science of soft-tissue healing, the adaptive changes of musculoskeletal and cardiovascular tissues as a result of conditioning and deconditioning, the influence of the central and peripheral nervous systems on motor behavior, and the functional anatomy of the area. Borrowing from all of these disciplines allows for the development of a treatment plan. This plan de-emphasizes a passive approach toward the management of low back disorders, and focuses instead on active restoration of function. The patient must recognize that he is ultimately responsible for managing his painful syndrome. The clinician then guides the patient through a phased rehabilitation process that is individually designed to maximize the potential for functional healing.

The purpose of this chapter is to detail the concepts and give examples of the methods used in each phase of the rehabilitation process for low back disorders. A phased rehabilitation program is dictated in part by the physiology of the tissues and the healing process. It should be recognized that vascularized tissues in any area of the body, whether they are contractile or noncontractile, have many similarities in regard to their physiology and their response to injury. The biomechanics and physiology of tissues in the low back are, therefore, similar to the biomechanics and physiology of tissues in other areas of the body. To view the low back differently invites treatment that is abstract and unscientific. The "mysticism" that potentially surrounds this type of approach results in the clinician's attempting to "heal the patient" rather than the patient managing his own complaint. More important, this type of

mismanagement often results in tissue dysfunction, frequent reinjury, and chronic symptoms.

This concept of low back treatment is not dissimilar to the management of any other mechanical musculoskeletal disorder. Once the clinician has the same level of understanding of the functional anatomy of the spine as he does of the functional anatomy of the peripheral joints, he can generate a treatment plan based on restoration of function. The focus is, therefore, on *function* rather than pain. Although pain cannot be ignored and certainly needs to be continually monitored and carefully evaluated by the clinician, it cannot be the primary focus of treatment.

It should be pointed out, however, that there is one important structure that is unique to the spine to which no comparison to the extremities can be made. That structure is the intervertebral disc. Mooney[13] suggests that because the healing potential of the intervertebral disc is different from that of other musculoskeletal tissues, perhaps it should be strongly suspected in that small group of patients with chronic and unrelenting pain, that is, those people who fail to respond in the time period normally allotted for adequate healing of other musculoskeletal tissues.

The essential health of the disc is maintained by a loading and unloading phenomena, and unchanging postures that result in a constant pressure, such as sitting, lying, or standing, lead to an interruption of pressure-dependent transfer of fluid. Thus even though the intervertebral disc may follow a different set of rules for healing when compared with other connective tissues of the body, passive therapeutic modalities and prolonged rest are not indicated for the intervertebral disc problem either; instead, the encouragement of function remains the primary goal.[13]

In order to present a rationale for the decision-making process behind the various therapeutic interventions for mechanical low back pain, we suggest that there are three major low back pain populations that can be targeted for goal-oriented rehabilitation emphasizing return to activity:

1. The acutely injured low back patient (acute injury).

2. The reinjury and/or exacerbation of a previous injury in a low back patient (reinjury syndrome).

3. The chronic low back pain patient (chronic pain syndrome).

In acute injury, the physical stimulus of injury bears a relatively straightforward relationship to the nociceptive response. The reinjury syndrome is that syndrome in which familiar symptoms and signs recur, usually as a result of activity or activities that cause an exacerbation of the patient's familiar problem. Lastly, in the chronic pain syndrome, the pain pattern becomes increasingly dissociated from the original physical mechanism of injury. Chronic pain and disability become more and more related to illness behavior and emotional distress than actual tissue damage.

It is important to note that "time" is not referred to in the definition of either the reinjury syndrome or the chronic pain syndrome. Both syndromes include people who have had low back pain over an extended period of time. However, the reinjury syndrome can involve exacerbations of previous injuries that perhaps have taken years to become symptomatic enough to cause the patient to seek help. Even though these exacerbations may occur over a very extended period of time, the patient does not have a significant behavioral component as the dominant feature and, by the above definitions, would not be considered a chronic pain patient. This fact is extremely important because the focus of treatment in the reinjury syndrome patient is significantly different from that in the chronic pain patient. More importantly, this thought process allows us to begin to separate the concept of low back pain from that of low back disability.

Distinction between the three types of syndromes is important because it provides more clear indications for using different therapeutic modalities. A significant low back pain population has been managed in the past with prolonged rest and repeated passive therapeutic interventions. Passive therapeutic interventions refer to the myriad of modalities, medications, and techniques that are applied to the patient by caregivers as opposed to the patient attempting to increase his own activity. The prolonged use of these types of interventions is inappropriate and has the potential to cause conversion of the acute injury or reinjury syndrome into a chronic pain syndrome. Their use can be indicated only for the initial stages of the acute injury syndrome or only occasionally for the initial stages of the reinjury syndrome. With continual use of these passive approaches, it is unreasonable to expect restoration of the patient to the preinjured state because of the inveterate catabolism that has already occurred.

Therefore, it is important to educate the patient at the outset that management of his lumbopelvic problem is ultimately his own responsibility. When this is recognized, reasonable goals can be set more easily. Likewise, delaying the effects of catabolism and ultimately training the neuromusculoskeletal system to better prepare the body to adapt to stresses placed on it take a much longer time than a few visits to the clinician's office. Within 2 weeks after an acute episode of low back pain, 50 per cent of patients recover, and after 1 month, 70 per cent recover.[9] Although 90 per cent of all low back problems spontaneously resolve after 3 months, 50 per cent of patients have recurrent episodes of low back pain.[1,10,23] Because recurrence is so common, the patient should ultimately be taught how to self-manage the problem. The therapist's role is to guide the patient through a program that assists with this goal.

THE IMPORTANCE OF BIOMECHANICAL COUNSELING

Before detailing the rehabilitation process, it is important to make some introductory comments regarding the concept of *biomechanical counseling*, since it helps to form the foundation of a rehabilitation program. Education in the form of biomechanical counseling becomes one of the most important aspects of a rehabilitation program. Because of its importance, it should be featured in all phases of the rehabilitation process. In its simplest form it is teaching the patient how to minimize the potential for nociceptive mechanical stresses to the injured area. Besides being an important first step in maximizing the potential for injured tissue to heal, it also initiates the process of having the patient become an active participant in his own rehabilitation program.

Why is the patient's active participation such an important component of rehabilitation? One of the primary reasons is due to a recognition of the amount of time a clinician actually interacts with a patient. If, for example, a patient is treated in a clinic three times a week for 45 minutes each session, this represents only 2 per cent of the time the patient is awake and resuming his activities of daily living! Therefore, to assume that three 45-minute treatments per week alone are going to significantly impact on the long-range outcome is unrealistic. Certainly there are isolated instances in which some mechanical low back disorders with a single causative incident completely respond with one or two treatments, never to recur. However, this does not seem to be the rule for the typical mechanical low back disorder seen in the average clinic.

The evaluation and assessment process described in Chapter 5 is the means to determine the information to be used for biomechanically counseling the patient. As discussed later in this chapter, the assessment provides the clinician with the information to determine the nociceptive biomechanics, and it is the individual counseling in the form of patient education that relates the individual patient's biomechanics of injury to his activities of daily living. Each patient has a unique set of limitations that can be determined only through a functional assessment. What might be a vulnerable position or movement for one patient's spine may not be a vulnerable position or movement for another patient's spine.

For this reason the "packaged" back school concepts can be effective for only a select group of patients whose unique problems fit the mechanics of that standardized program. It is unreasonable and often impossible to teach all patients to maintain one particular spinal position. These programs make the assumption that all patients have the same functional limitations, and that their mechanics of injury and pain reproduction are similar. Because they are seldom comparable, such programs can

only be expected to assist in the management of a select group of patients.

INJURY, THE HEALING PROCESS, AND RESTORATION OF FUNCTION: A COMPARISON WITH THE TREATMENT APPROACH TO THE EXTREMITIES

Injury processes and the responses of the tissue to injury are discussed in Chapter 1. Likewise, the repair of tissues as a result of injury is covered earlier in this text. With this background, it might be appropriate to now compare the treatment philosophy for the lumbopelvic region with that for the extremities.

There are two main reasons why injury to the low back parallels injury to the extremities. First, as in the extremities, it is unreasonable to think that only one isolated structure becomes injured. For example, the joints, discs, muscles, and connective tissue structures of the spine do not act in isolation, but rather work in concert with one another in the attenuation and transference of forces, much like the capsule, intra- and extra-articular ligaments, and muscles of the joints of the extremities. Injury to any one component alters function of the remaining structures.[17,18]

Second, scar tissue, which is so important for the repair process, is not an exact match of the tissue that was injured. The healing process for the low back is similar to that for the rest of the body. Injured tissue is repaired by the formation of granulation and scar tissue.[6,7,24,28] Consequently the function of tissues in the postinjury state is different from that in the preinjury state.

Even though a comparison between knee injuries and low back injuries has been made in Chapter 1, further discussion is warranted in regard to a practical rehabilitation philosophy. A suitable clinical example is the anterior cruciate ligament disorder of the knee. Once this ligament is torn or sprained to a degree that its viscoelastic properties have been changed, function of the knee is permanently altered. The person will never have a "normal" knee again, no matter how precise the surgical repair or how comprehensive the rehabilitation. The clinician's role in this case is to rehabilitate the knee in order to allow the patient to optimally manage his activities, recognizing that a return to the preinjury state is highly unlikely. In short, the patient may need to modify his activities in order to accommodate to this problem. The clinician, recognizing the mechanics of injury, can show the patient different movements or activities that may reinjure the area. In addition, the clinician designs a rehabilitation program that helps to train the neuromuscular and musculoskeletal systems to keep the injured tissue away from the upper limits of its physiologic tolerances.

The same rationale should be used for the lumbopelvic region. Once any major tissues of this area are sprained, strained, or torn because of injury, their function is permanently altered. This injury in turn alters the mechanics of the surrounding tissues. As with rehabilitation of the anterior cruciate ligament injury, the goal of rehabilitation is to teach the patient how to manage his problem and learn the limits of his activities. This is a logical approach, since torn and subsequently repaired tissue has reduced load-bearing capabilities, whether that load be applied in the form of compression, tension, torsion, or shear.

There are certainly exceptions to the discussion above regarding patient management. For example, isolated sacroiliac joint pain might be seen in multiparous women, especially as a result of childbirth. Subluxation of the joint might occur if forces exceed the capacity of the stabilizing tissues. If this is the case, mobilization or manipulation of the joint followed by external support of the region in the form of an orthosis may offer dramatic relief.

Another example of immediate relief for a mechanical low back problem occurs during the abdominal and low back postural changes of pregnancy. These may result in excessive stress being placed on otherwise normal low back tissues, such as the zygapophysial joints structures, owing to the change in the location of the weight line as it traverses the lumbopelvic tissues. To accommodate this altered weight line, a lumbar support in the form of an orthosis might provide a counterforce that helps to redirect the weight line and marginally unload the soft tissues so that the painful stimulus can be diminished.

The two examples above are mentioned to recognize that a clinical intervention might result in changing the patient's pain pattern quickly, dramatically, and perhaps permanently. This is certainly the exception rather than the rule with the most common low back problems. In these more common clinical syndromes the history is extended over a greater period of time, and the patient presents with a problem that features a number of acute episodes of a chronic syndrome. Directing therapy toward the neuromuscular system to encourage the restoration of function is the goal with such patients.

AGE-RELATED CHANGES VERSUS SOFT-TISSUE SPRAINS AND STRAINS

Since Mixter and Barr's[12] classic work in regard to the potential of the intervertebral disc to "rupture," there has been a great deal of focus on disc pathology as a primary source of low back pain. By contrast, the potential for soft tissues of the low back (strains and sprains) to result in low back pain has received much less attention. Sprain and strain of the low back as a mechanism for low back pain is not as readily accepted as the intervertebral disc lesion. This is surprising, since the natural course of resolution for a low back injury (90 per cent will resolve within 3 months—see above) fits very well within time constraints required for resolution of soft-tissue injuries elsewhere in the body.

Great advances have also been made in diagnostic radiology. As a result, the basis for many diagnoses is structural pathology. Because disc bulges or degenerative joint disease of the spine can easily be seen with imaging techniques, whereas soft-tissue injuries cannot, it is easy to dismiss soft tissues as being responsible for low back pain. However, this is not justified, since the physiologic responses of low back soft tissues owing to excessive forces should be identical to those of soft tissues elsewhere in the body.

In reality, the picture gained from the various imaging techniques presents a view of the aging process of the spine, which may or may not be relevant to the problem. However, because the diagnostic picture is seen at the same time that the person presents himself in clinic with his complaint, it is certainly tempting to consider basing the diagnosis on this structural condition. Structural changes, however, often do not present any symptoms. Weisel and coworkers[26] demonstrated this quite readily in their Volvo Award paper reviewing computed tomography scans of the lumbar region. Although disc bulges were diagnosed in a large number of the reports, the patient in fact was asymptomatic. The same misinterpretation of the relation between structural changes and symptoms might occur with any radiograph that reveals the normal aging process. Further work must be done in order to clarify the difference between age-related changes and true pathologic changes.

Finally, it is quite apparent that complaints of low back pain peak during the middle-age years and subsequently decline as the person ages. This does not correlate with the natural process of spine degeneration. If structural pathology were responsible for the majority of low back syndromes, we should expect that low back pain would peak in the later years and correlate more closely to age-related changes seen in the spine. It does not, so it behooves us to give strong consideration to other sources of pain in the spine.

INTENT OF TREATMENT

Before proceeding into the objectives and phases of rehabilitation for lumbopelvic disorders, the intent of treatment should be stated. The intent of treatment of the lumbopelvic region has the same guidelines as for other areas of the body, and can be summarized as follows:

1. To optimize the healing environment

2. To restore anatomical relations between injured and noninjured tissue

3. To maintain the normal function of non-injured tissues

4. To prevent excessive strain from being put on injured tissue

This summary of the intent of treatment for the healing of collagen structures was first presented by van der Muelen.[24] It can easily be applied to the treatment of lumbopelvic disorders.

Optimization of Healing Environment

The first component of the intent of treatment relates to the clinician's ability to optimize the healing environment in order to give the wound a chance to heal. Although "wound" may conjure up thoughts of skin lacerations, torn tissue, and bleeding, this concept should be extended to include any tissue, superficial or deep, in which the structural makeup of cells or fibers has been altered by injury. We subscribe to the premise that there is a potential for the muscles, tendons, ligaments, fascia, or any tissue in the lumbopelvic region to be injured, in addition to the intervertebral disc and zygapophyseal joints. The injury may be, for example, a sprain of the annulus fibrosus, the iliolumbar ligament, or the zygapophyseal joint capsule, or strain of the iliocostalis lumborum or multifidus muscle. The injury probably involves several tissues. No matter which tissues are involved, the initial goal of management in each case remains maximizing the wound-healing potential.

The sports medicine literature is replete with information concerning soft-tissue injury of the extremities, and it is beyond the scope of this text to list and discuss various soft-tissue injuries. It is a well-accepted fact, however, that sprain and strain are the most common and often disabling injuries of athletes. McMaster's[11] classic work on muscle-tendon injury and Noyes and colleagues'[16] landmark work with stress-strain rates of ligament injuries have markedly enhanced our understanding of these common clinical problems. They also have provided valid evaluation tests and treatment interventions for muscular and ligamentous injuries of the peripheral joints. As we increase our understanding of the functional anatomy of the low back, especially in regard to the large forces that the tissues are subject to, it is reasonable to conclude that the same type of injuries that occur in the extremities can occur in any tissue of the spine. However, without the technology to measure such injury, this remains to be validated.

The real question that the clinician must answer in this first intent of treatment is how to maximize the ability of the body to, quite literally, heal itself. Therein lies one of the major dilemmas in dealing with low back disorders. It is hard to create an environment that allows for strong functional healing because of the difficulty in balancing rest with activity in the lumbopelvic region. Optimally we would like to position the region in such a way that it provides the appropriate environment for wound-healing. However, because it is the hub of weight-bearing (Chapter 1), this is difficult to do.

The low back cannot be immobilized like the extremities, so close attention to the results of the assessment is required in order to determine the forces that reproduce the patient's familiar symptoms. This is an important distinction between performing a low back evaluation to identify a particular tissue at fault versus performing an evaluation to assess the stresses that reproduce familiar pain. Biomechanical counseling becomes an exercise in teaching the patient how these nociceptive biomechanics relate to his activities of daily living. In order to allow for wound-healing and to optimize the healing environment, whether it be an acute injury or an acute exacerbation of a chronic injury, this aspect is crucial to an understanding of the sensible management of low back pain.

Restoration of Anatomical Relations Between Injured and Noninjured Tissue

As soon as possible after injury, controlled nondestructive motions must be properly introduced into the area so that the injured tissues will heal according to appropriate stress lines. Tissues must also be free to glide over, compress onto, and apply tension to surrounding tissues. In short, tissues interact with their surrounding tissues. It is necessary that they begin to heal in a manner that does not alter the function of surrounding tissues.

Injury to tissues results in a cascade of events that proceed sequentially and include phases that start with the inflammatory process and culminate in a repair that ideally allows for nondestructive movement patterns of the injured region. Nikolaou and associates[15] present evidence of the speed with which muscle repair occurs using animal models. In these studies contractile ability of the muscle decreased consistently by 70 per cent immediately after injury, while the degree of edema was maximal during the first 24 hours. After 48 hours recovery of the muscle's mechanical functions began to occur even though there was still marked inflammation and fibroblastic activity. By one week after injury the mechanical function of muscle had returned to 92 per cent of the controls, but scarring and fibrosis were noted. The cascade of events thus proceed quite rapidly.

Maintenance of Normal Function of Noninjured Tissue

Care must be taken to maintain the health and strength of the various tissues, with specific attention given to preventing the effects of disuse and altered motor behavior. A phased treatment program allows for early mobilization and recognizes the important balance necessary between activity and wound-healing.

The strong argument for early mobilization is in agreement with the data that has accumulated regarding the appropriate length of time for bed rest after the low back injury. There is good evidence to suggest that longer than 48 hours is counterproductive and contributes to the catabolic, deconditioning changes seen in the chronic back patient who has been mismanaged (Chapter 1).

Early mobilization of the region is, therefore, extremely important for successful management. Prolonging the immobilization and bed rest periods for most mechanical soft-tissue injuries invites weakening of the connective tissue structures, loss of muscle and bone strength, decreased cardiovascular efficiency, and altered neurotrophic function, such as incoordination.

Prevention of Excessive Stress on Injured Tissue

This intent requires knowledge of the basic science of tissue-healing and the biomechanics of the lumbopelvic region. It necessitates starting a training program that does not continually disrupt the healing process. Training is important because the lumbopelvic tissues must ultimately accept the various stresses to which they are subjected, but it must be done in a manner that does not cause reinjury. The results of mismanagement are compromised function, frequent reinjury, with resulting chronic symptoms.

OBJECTIVES OF TREATMENT

There are five broad objectives to be considered in the treatment of mechanical low back pain. These objectives relate directly to the three target populations for intervention referred to earlier. Details of a treatment plan to carry out these objectives is provided below in the section on Phases of Treatment.

The first objective is pain modulation or promotion of analgesia. Various modalities and pharmacologic agents are effective for this objective and are certainly indicated for the acutely injured low back patient and occasionally for the acute exacerbation of the patient with the reinjury syndrome. In both cases, they should be used sparingly and over a minimal time period. They are usually not indicated in the chronic pain syndrome.

The second objective is biomechanical counseling. The details of this process have already been described. It should be evident that this objective is most indicated for the reinjury syndrome. Certainly when the acutely injured patient has decreased symptoms, this objective becomes an important consideration.

The third objective is to begin to generate controlled forces into a region in order to promote nondestructive movements. The phases

of treatment describe techniques that can be used to generate these forces. The result of meeting this objective is to affect fluid dynamics, increase afferent input into the nervous system (which modulates pain and reflexively alters the resting state of muscle tonus), and modify connective tissue. This objective is most indicated in the reinjury syndrome. Because most of the techniques are passive ones, they are rarely indicated for the chronic pain patient.

The fourth objective is to enhance neuromuscular efficiency. This objective encourages activity and is met through the application of various types of training, strengthening, and neuromuscular reeducation programs. These programs are effective because the training effects to the muscles augment force attenuation capabilities, and patterns of movement are taught that are meant to minimize mechanical stress. It is especially indicated for the reinjury syndrome and the chronic pain syndrome. Meeting this objective is especially important for the chronic pain patient since the emphasis for this patient is always on increasing activity and measuring this increase in function in order to make patients aware of these positive changes in their activity levels.

The fifth objective is to establish limits. Although detailed below, it is important to note how important this is for all three types of patients. When this objective is met, the patient develops a better understanding of his physical limitations and recognizes that he is ultimately responsible for staying within those constraints.

PHASES OF TREATMENT

We have divided the treatment protocol into four phases for ease of discussion (Fig. 6–1). There are many modes of treatment for lumbopelvic disorders. We present a systematic overview of the phases that allow many of the techniques currently used to be classified under one or more phases.

Why should this effort be undertaken? We subscribe to the philosophy that there are many ways to significantly impact on a pa-

REHABILITATION PROCESS PHASES I-IV

PHASE I

- Treatment of pain
  - Modalities
  - Medication
- Support the region (rest)
- Biomechanical counseling (rest)

PHASE II

- Continue support
- Begin nondestructive movement
  - Generate afferent input
    - Passive
    - Active
- Biomechanical counseling (decrease the destructive behavior)

PHASE III

- Discontinue support
- Begin *proprioceptive and kinesthetic strength training* in a protected range (unshaded area)
  - Neuromuscular efficiency
  - Dynamic stabilization

PHASE IV

- Establishment of limits
  - Movement
  - Loads
  - Positions
  - Frequencies

Figure 6–1. *Four phases of rehabilitation. The patient does not have to begin with phase one, but can enter the system in any one of the phases. He may revert back to the initial phase if an exacerbation of symptoms occurs during the rehabilitation program.*

late that the nervous system is the key component being affected, although explanations of successful management are routinely attributed to influences on the connective and muscle tissues. The concept of neuromodulation resulting from treatment is discussed below.

Phase One

Phase one is the period when pain is treated, and initiating steps to optimize the healing environment becomes the most important consideration. This phase poses a dilemma for the clinician. Pain must be acknowledged and certainly respected, yet it cannot be the focus of the rehabilitation process. A delicate balance between treating the pain and preparing the patient for recovery must be achieved so that the clinician can commence with a more active intervention.

In order to institute effective pain management the clinician should begin to educate the patient about the importance of recognizing pain patterns, especially if one of the desired outcomes of a rehabilitation process is to teach the patient how to ultimately cope with his own low back problem. The patient needs to understand the importance of recognizing changes in intensity, frequency, and duration of pain. Combinations of these elements result in a pain pattern. The clinician should try to increase the patient's sensitivity to any of these changes because so often the patient acknowledges only intensity. Successful management of pain by the clinician or the patient results if there is favorable alteration of any of the components of the pain pattern. The clinician must take the time to educate the patient, since the more the patient understands, the easier and more successful will be the long-term rehabilitation outcome.

The clinician has many therapeutic options available to deal effectively with the patient's pain. Physical agents, such as thermomodalities and electromodalities, are often used in combination with medications. They promote analgesia, inhibit an exuberant inflammatory process, and decrease the muscle spasm that typically accompanies injury. It is entirely eth-

tient's pain or function. Rather than focus on the techniques, we believe that it is more important to analyze how the particular technique is influencing the neuromusculoskeletal system. In essence, there are common denominators of the many and varied approaches to treatment. Certainly many are successful, albeit by anecdotal evidence. The common denominator, however, may be the influence on the neuromusculoskeletal system. We specu-

ical and indeed the clinician's responsibility to use these forms of treatment during this initial phase. However, their limits must be recognized. There is no evidence that they greatly accelerate the cellular aspects of the healing process.[7] Rather, they enable the clinician to move the patient quickly toward increased activity, and allow the early introduction of nondestructive forces into the injured region.

Prolonged use of physical agents and medications leads to patient dependency on these interventions, and potentially transfers the responsibility of management from the patient to the clinician. If medications and a specific physical agent are used initially to decrease pain in order to allow return to activity, then their use is justified. It is in the patient's best interest, however, if they are used sparingly and briefly.

A comment regarding the use of the various physical agents and medications to decrease inflammation is also in order. Inflammation is a normal process of healing, and careful consideration should be given as to whether it needs to be discouraged. The chemical environment resulting from inflammation initiates the activation of the nociceptor system, which in turn gives rise to the subjective experience of pain (Chapter 2). In order that a pain behavior have less of a chance to develop, it is certainly important to control inflammation, and thus pain. This is one reason modalities or medications may have their place. However, recognizing the time frames for the inflammatory process, it should be apparent that extensive, long-term use of modalities or medications is entirely unjustified and contributes to patient dependency.

Another indication for the use of specific physical agents or medications is if the intent of treatment is to decrease stasis or fluid accumulation. Some modalities, such as electrical stimulation that results in muscle contraction, facilitate fluid dynamics, while other physical agents or medications change the frequency, intensity, or duration of pain to allow active movements by the patient. Active movement facilitates fluid dynamics and promotes the elimination of stasis by helping to flush fluid from the injured area.

The first phase of treatment also includes rest for the injured area. However, the term *rest* has led to misconceptions regarding its use in the management of mechanical disorders of the low back. Rest refers to minimizing the opportunities for forces to accumulate in the injured area—trying to keep the region invulnerable. It does not necessarily mean bed rest; in fact, bed rest is counterproductive to the effective management of mechanical low back disorders. Unless the patient is appropriately biomechanically counseled, he will be unable to keep the area at rest, since the low back is the hub of weight-bearing into which the trunk and ground forces converge (Chapter 1). Biomechanical counseling is thus one of the most important aspects of the first phase of treatment. Keeping the area at rest refers to the maintenance of activity while at the same time improving the patient's ability to keep destructive forces away from the injured tissue.

This concept of rest needs to be analyzed in greater detail to underscore why the evaluation system discussed in Chapter 5 is so important. In order to help with an understanding of this concept, the reader is referred to Figure 6–2, which represents a hypothetical center of pressure from a line of weight-bearing. Movement by the patient causes this line of weight-bearing to traverse different regions of the lumbopelvic region. For descriptive purposes, the line of weight-bearing is shown traversing the lumbar spine. The square is used to signify the boundaries of the area through which the weight-bearing line moves as a result of motion of the lumbar spine.

As the weight-bearing line, represented by the arrow, moves through the square representing the potential motion area of that segment, the tissues of the spine that surround the line experience various forces, such as compression, tension, shear, and torsion. As an example of a relatively straightforward circumstance, forward bending causes the weight-bearing line to migrate anteriorly. Tissues anterior to this line may have more compressive force applied to them than before the forward bending movement, while there is increased tensile force on posterior tissues. The complexity of analyzing the forces increases when we begin to add multiplanar motion as well as the elements of muscle contraction to

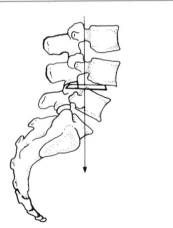

Figure 6–2. Three-dimensional square representing the range of motion in which a weight line or center of pressure travels. This hypothetical window can be placed between the fourth and fifth lumbar vertebrae, and the arrow is in the center as the patient is standing erect. The front portion represents anterior, the back portion represents posterior, the right represents the right side, and the left represents the left side.

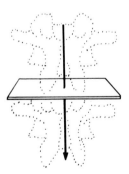

Figure 6–3. Clear box indicates painless, full range of motion.

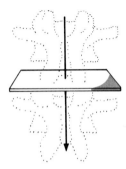

Figure 6–4. Hypothetical window with shaded area representing a noxious or destructive stimulus as the weight line enters this region. In this example backward bending and side bending to the right produces the familiar pain and results in a noxious or destructive stimulus.

the moving segment. It is impossible to measure the forces. Instead, the attempt is to focus on the directions and types of force.

The clear box represents the painless motion permitted (Fig. 6–3). The shaded area (Fig. 6–4) represents the findings of the assessment, that is, the determination of those forces and movements that stimulate the nociceptive system of this region and cause the familiar pain experienced by the patient. (Hereafter in this chapter the region in which familiar pain is elicited is referred to as the shaded area.) In other words, motions that the patient performs, or the passive movements imparted by the clinician, should be analyzed as to both the movement patterns and the resulting forces that are reaching the region and stimulating the nociceptive system.

In the example shown in Figure 6–4 one can see that backward bending combined with side bending to the right is the motion that reproduces the painful pattern. More specifically, this motion brings the weight-bearing line toward the right posterolateral corner of the motion "window" and signifies the area that must be initially avoided in the movement portion of the treatment program. Note, however, that there are many ways to introduce these same forces and movements into the right posterolateral corner besides backward bending and side bending to the right. The pushoff phase of gait on the right lower extremity, reaching overhead to pull an object off a shelf, walking or running downhill, sitting with a pillow in the lumbar region forcing the spine into hyperextension, or even a prone yoga position in

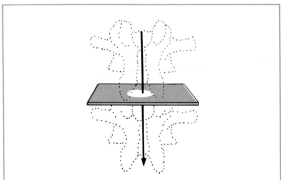

Figure 6–5. Window representing a patient who has only limited nondestructive range of motion within which to move without reinjury.

which the person is arching the lumbar spine by pushing up with his hands all place similar forces through this "window."

Figure 6–5 shows another example of a patient who, as a result of a particular movement pattern, stimulates the nociceptive system, which reproduces his familiar complaint. In this example, however, the patient has only a limited nondestructive range of motion within which to move without reinjury.

In order to begin early mobilization the clinician must realize these nociceptive biomechanics and avoid the shaded area in the treatment process. Each person's painful region is unique, yet it is important to identify this region, since it is impossible to initially rest the injured area and begin a strong healing process if the area is continuously provoked.

Resting the region may also necessitate altering the way in which forces reach this area. A clinical example is a frontal plane asymmetry of pelvic position in which the left side of the pelvis is lower than the right. This finding might be caused by skeletal differences and neuromuscular imbalances in the musculature responsible for the frontal plane position of the pelvis. The outcome is an asymmetrical weight-bearing pattern of tissues in the lumbopelvic region owing to the lateral pelvic tilt downward on the left and the resultant lumbar side bending to the right (Fig. 6–6). Note how this standing posture of the lumbopelvic region results in the weight-bearing line (referred to

above and in Fig. 6–4) also traversing the right posterolateral corner of the "window" in the lumbar spine. From the perspective of force analysis, the convergence of forces into the region with this particular frontal plane asymmetry produces a fairly similar accumulation of forces to the lumbar spine as do backward bending and side bending to the right. Certainly the magnitude of the forces is not exactly equal, nor is the direction. What is more important, however, is that both scenarios have the potential to load the same area in much the same manner and minimize the potential for functional healing. In order to successfully manage these nociceptive mechanics, the frontal plane position must be changed in order to help unload the injured region.

A short discourse regarding the accumulation of forces through the lumbopelvic region owing to an asymmetrical frontal plane is warranted to underscore how important it is to

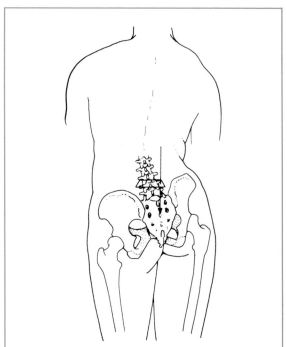

Figure 6–6. Left frontal plane asymmetry that shifts the center of pressure or compressive force to the right posterior aspect of the window.

minimize these forces during the first phase of treatment. Note how the standing frontal plane asymmetry causes various mechanical changes. The right posterolateral aspect of the lumbosacral intervertebral disc has increased compression on the right, the right intervertebral foramen of the lumbar spine is narrowed, the right lumbosacral zygapophyseal joint is in the closed-packed position, and the contractile tissues of the lumbar spine on the right are in a shortened position and lengthened on the left. At the pelvis the right sacroiliac joint has an increased shear force to it, while the left realizes more of a compressive force as compared with the symmetrical anatomic position (Fig. 6–7).

The hip joints are also affected by this frontal plane asymmetry. The right femur adopts a relatively adducted position with respect to the pelvis, and the left femur is relatively abducted. This position potentially results in altered weight-bearing patterns of the hip. At the right hip joint there is an increased vertical force to the femoral head, while at the left hip joint there is an increased bending movement at the femoral neck. The lateral musculature of the right hip will be contracting from an elongated position, and the musculature of the left

hip will be contracting from a relatively shortened position (Fig. 6–7). The significance to this shift of forces throughout the lumbopelvic region with a frontal plane asymmetry is potential compressive, tensile, and shear overload to various tissues. This increases the chances for the propagation of tissue irritation and the prolongation of symptoms.

One relatively simple way to manage this condition during the initial phase of treatment is by using a heel lift, which may help to centralize the line of gravity through the tissues by altering the frontal plane position of the pelvis (Fig. 6–8). This in itself may be considered a form of rest for any of the aforementioned tissues that might be injured from overload. The trunk and ground forces now converge on the various lumbopelvic tissues in a more symmetrical, less destructive manner. More likely the injured tissue is slightly unloaded, which helps to optimize the healing environment for the injured tissue. Balancing the weight-bearing line in this manner is often a valuable adjunct during the initial phases of tissue healing, especially if the patient responds favorably to the correction during the evaluation process.

These temporary lifts can be fabricated by using Corex cork, Spenco, and Barge glue. The technique involves cutting the desired shape to fit the heel of the shoe out of the thickness of cork (⅛ in, ¼ in, ⅜ in). The usual thickness is one half of the discrepancy noted in the standing evaluation. The reason to start with this height is to gradually apply the new forces into the axial skeleton, especially if the person is extremely active. A lift that is thicker than ⅜ in raises the heel out of the shoe's counter and usually cannot be tolerated within the shoe. The surfaces of the cork and the Spenco are glued together, and a grinder is used to bevel the front edge. Once the heel lift has been determined to be effective, it can be incorporated into an orthotic.

During this initial phase a lumbar or sacroiliac orthosis can also be used to help stabilize and support the area, and thus improve conditions for healing. Stabilization probably results from the cutaneous input the orthosis provides, which contributes to proprioceptive and kinesthetic awareness of spine position

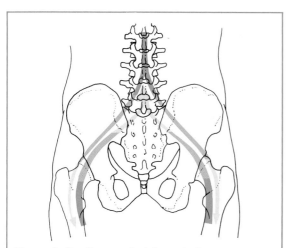

Figure 6–7. Symmetrical frontal plane representing a shared compressive and shear force by both sacroiliac joints.

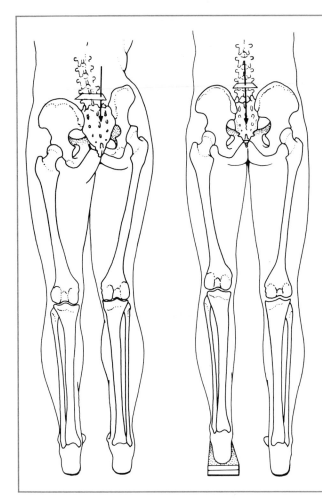

Figure 6–8. Heel lift used under the left lower extremity to balance the frontal plane of the skeleton, and in essence resting the region and moving the center of pressure away from the noxious stimulus.

and movement. Figures 6–9 and 6–10 show examples of lumbar and sacroiliac orthoses. The orthosis cannot be expected to completely immobilize the area. However, the increased afferent input to the central nervous system in combination with the external support increases awareness of lumbopelvic position and motion.

Phase Two

During phase two the clinician initiates techniques that provide afferent input into the central nervous system by way of the application of forces into and around the injured area. Early, nondestructive movement or forces are introduced into the injured region, which is advantageous to the functional healing process.

The application of forces or movements has a threefold intent. First, the tissue is stimulated along appropriate stress lines. The intent is to direct forces to the injured tissues in a nondestructive manner in order to stimulate the orientation of collagen in a functional pattern. Second, the important afferent component of the neurologic system is activated, which has the potential to modulate pain as well as provide proprioceptive input to the central ner-

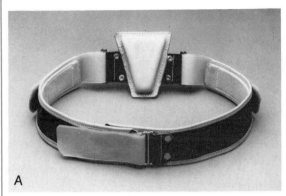

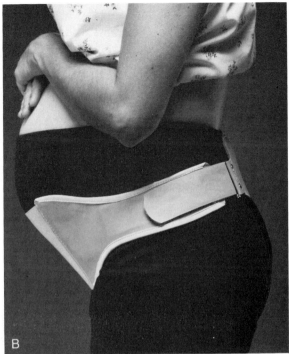

Figure 6–9. *A*, Sacral support used to create a posterior-to-anterior force of the sacrum and a posterior rotary movement to the ilium as the belt is tightened. This support is made of leather and a viscoelastic polymer that is designed to be anatomically compatible and create the previously mentioned forces into and through the pelvis. (IEM Orthopaedics, P.O. Box 592, Ravenna, Ohio 44266)

B, Adaptation of the sacral component adapted for the pregnant population. This *uses* an anterior window of elastic that allows the belt to conform to the abdomen. Posterior view *C* shows placement of the triangular pad on the sacrum. (IEM Orthopaedics, P.O. Box 592, Ravenna, Ohio 44266)

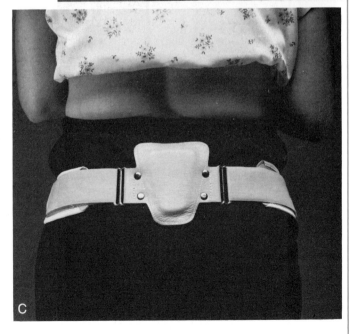

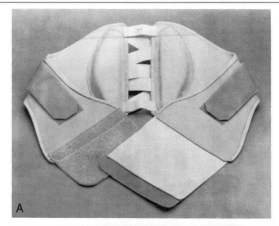

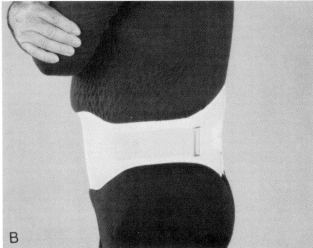

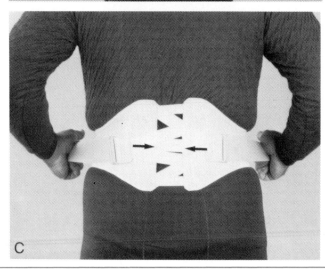

Figure 6–10. *A–C,* Lumbar support based on a patented securing and tightening system designed to create a resultant force of compressing the posterior lumbar tissues into the lamina and spinous process of the vertebral bodies. This support is tightened from the side and can be easily loosened to fit the needs of the patient. (IEM Orthopaedics, P.O. Box 592, Ravenna, Ohio 44266)

vous system.[27] Third, forces and movements enhance fluid dynamics.

The intensity, frequency, and duration of this manual aspect of the treatment process depends on the technique chosen as well as the skill of the clinician in recognizing the potential for exacerbation of the injury. Being too aggressive in this phase prolongs the inflammatory process of the injured tissues.

Therefore, the clinician is faced with the decision of how much is enough and how much is too much, recognizing that the ultimate goal with this rehabilitation philosophy is an early return to activity with an emphasis on function. Active and active assistive manual treatment must be provided carefully to strike a balance between therapeutic recovery and avoidance of reinjury. The clinician is also faced with the dilemma of determining when, or if ever, the techniques should be done in a manner that begins to approach the painful movement pattern. The movement aspects of the treatment process should first be carried out in the invulnerable range of the movement pattern that was determined during the standing examination.

Once the healing process has begun, the clinician must make a clinical judgment as to the extent to which the shaded area can be infiltrated. Depending on the severity of the injury, this area may or may not be approached without further exacerbation of the syndrome. Unfortunately no specific criteria are available to make this judgment, and the clinician relies on past experience and his reassessment skills to render this determination.

The reality of some low back problems is that the patient has significantly injured tissues of the spine, and they will never be able to painlessly enter this shaded region that represents their vulnerable spine mechanics. Therefore, the patient and the clinician must accept this fact, and both must devise alternative strategies to carry out a specific task. This is no different than the clinical strategy used for the patient with a severe anterior cruciate ligament injury to the knee or a chronic, frequently provoked tendinitis. Pain that comes and promptly leaves is acceptable; however, pain that remains for hours or days after treatment may indicate excessive aggressiveness.

Unfortunately the patient's activities of daily living also contribute to the propagation of pain; therefore, a careful evaluation of these activities and their influence on provocation of the syndrome must be assessed before treatment by the clinician is incriminated.

If an exacerbation occurs, the treatment process can be redirected to the first phase. This exacerbation is not necessarily unfavorable. The clinician and the patient can use this information to redefine the status of the injured tissues and can use this time to educate the patient as to the mechanics of the reinjury in the controlled environment of the clinic. If the goal is to educate the patient as to the management of his low back syndrome, an exacerbation of the familiar injury in such a controlled environment can be invaluable in the education process.

Although this second phase is important, it cannot be the final phase. Often treatment is prolonged throughout this phase, or stops after the patient's pain is lessened. This type of narrowed thought process often contributes to the chronicity of lumbopelvic problems. Rather than directing the rehabilitation process toward the restoration of function, the focus is solely on decreasing pain. We subscribe to the philosophy that this second phase, as well as phase one, has the ultimate goal of expeditiously preparing the patient for the training phases (phases three and four) of the rehabilitation process. The active remodeling of tissue by means of a training program is needed to assure the development of the tissues' ability to withstand the forces of daily activity without reinjury. Passive treatment processes and the do-something-to-me attitude of the patient do not represent a means to an end with respect to assuring an active, relatively pain-free lifestyle.

There are a variety of ways in which the clinician can introduce passive and active assistive nondestructive forces into the tissues. Although these techniques have different names and often purport to be entirely unique, they have a great deal of commonality. Effective techniques to introduce nondestructive forces into the region, to promote fluid dynamics, and to increase afferent input into the central nervous system include joint mobilization, soft-tissue mobilization, massage, manipulation, traction, muscle energy, prolonged stretching, transverse friction, acupressure, myofascial techniques, and contract-relax techniques.

Whether we are "repositioning" bones in such an inherently stable complex as the lumbopelvic region, reducing a subluxation of joints, or altering the neuromuscular physiology and mechanics of connective tissue is certainly open for question. It is our opinion that the unifying theme and ultimate result of these and other manual techniques are that forces are placed on tissues and joints, and that these forces increase afferent input to the central nervous system. This afferent input sets the balance of motor activity necessary for proper transferral of the forces of gravity and movement. With this new neuromuscular set as a major outcome of the treatment, it is easy to understand why such a variety of techniques can all be successful in this phase.

The bases for the techniques should be the

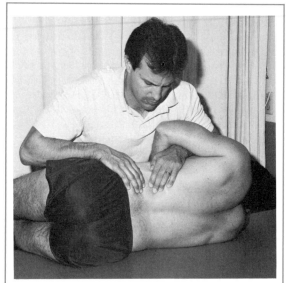

Figure 6–12. One of many soft-tissue mobilization techniques designed to assist in fluid dynamics as well as affecting the afferent system.

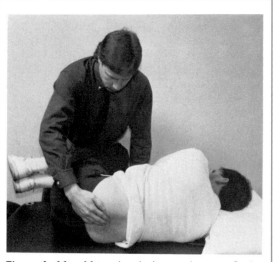

Figure 6–11. Manual technique to impart a flexion and an extension force to the lumbar spine in a side lying position. The clinician can use the femurs as a lever to impart nondestructive forces to the lumbar tissues. In this example the patient's knees are flexed and the clinician is controlling the patient's femurs with his body and at the same time using his hands to control the forces to the lumbar spine.

understanding of the functional anatomy of the spine and the desired outcome of the force generated to the region. Anytime the clinician directs a force to the body he should be able to visualize that force into and through the anatomical structures, and relate that force to the overall goals of this phase.

Some of these techniques warrant further comments regarding their use. Massage—in particular effleurage—soft-tissue mobilization, joint mobilization, and myofascial techniques can all theoretically minimize fluid stasis, and their potential effectiveness should not be overlooked. Figure 6–11 shows flexion and extension lumbar joint mobilization being imparted to the lumbar spine by the clinician. It is easy to appreciate the potential of this technique to affect fluid dynamics. Figure 6–12 shows methods of mobilizing the soft tissue in order to assist with fluid dynamics.

Various techniques also have the effect of stimulating the articular mechanoreceptors, muscle proprioceptors, and cutaneous receptors. The effects of this increased afferent input include pain modulation and the initiation of reflex responses of the motor program centers in the spinal cord and supraspinal regions. Soft-tissue mobilization, joint mobilization, and myofascial techniques, as well as muscle energy, stretching of lumbar tissues, manual traction, and manipulation to the lumbar spine, all potentially increase afferent input to the central nervous system. Figure 6–13 shows transverse friction to deep tissues in the lumbosacral triangle.[4] Figure 6–14 shows myofascial techniques that can effectively stimulate the receptor system. Figure 6–15 shows muscle energy techniques that increase afferent input owing to stimulation of the muscle proprioceptors, as well as the application of forces to the joints by means of isometric muscle contraction. Figure 6–16 shows the application of a manual traction force to the lumbar spine, and Figure 6–17 shows and describes a typical position for manipulation.

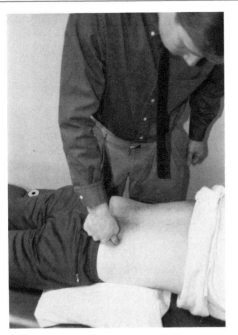

Figure 6–13. Deep transverse friction massage at the lumbosacral triangle.

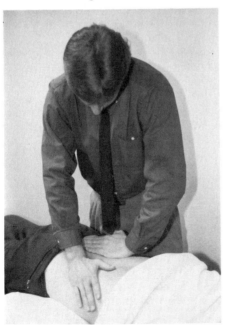

Figure 6–14. Technique that effectively stimulates the receptors through hands on mobilization of the dermal and myofascial systems.

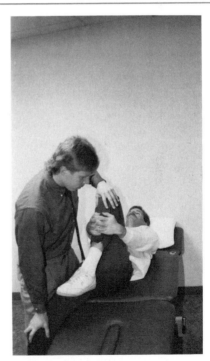

Figure 6–15. Muscle energy technique used to create an anterior force to the right ilium and a posterior force to the left ilium.

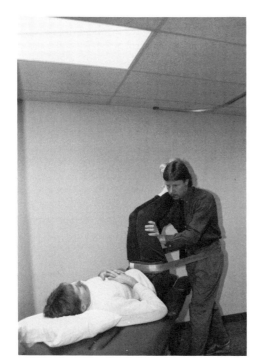

Figure 6–16. Manually produced traction force to the lumbar spine.

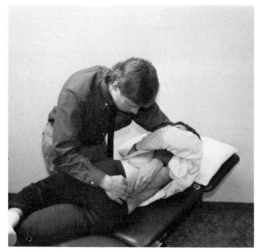

Figure 6–17. Positioning the patient in left lumbar rotation so that mobilizations can be performed.

There is certainly some question as to whether these techniques "reposition" bones, reduce subluxation, reposition disc fragments, or "release" connective tissue to the extent that intertissue and intratissue movements are now facilitated. We are skeptical that any of these purported results occur in the majority of instances. What appears to be a more reasonable explanation, based on known neuromuscular physiology, is a resultant change in the neuromuscular set of the surrounding region owing to application of the technique. This change by means of neuromodulation ultimately affects movement patterns and the subjective pain experience. However, this remains to be experimentally proven.

What is more important to consider is that although the application of these forces into the region remains extremely important during this phase, the clinician should realize that at this time the injury site is undergoing a remodeling phase of the healing process.[7,24,28] With this in mind, techniques should be chosen not only for their efficacy in modulating pain and altering the neuromuscular set, but also to minimize the chance of reintroducing the same destructive forces that were gleaned from the evaluation.

For example, the goal of the clinician might be to place stretching or lengthening forces on left lumbosacral musculature that travel superiorly, anteriorly, and medially (i.e., the quadratus lumborum and deep erector spinae). The patient could be positioned in a right side lying position, over a rolled pillow or bolster (Fig. 6–18). The clinician faces the patient and manually controls the contract-relax-stretch maneuver. The stretch force can be released, and the patient can be asked to contract against a small resistance. The stretch is then repeated.

This technique of stretching the lumbar musculature is very effective, but the clinician must realize that the position of the lumbopelvic region and the forces related to the stretch potentially make other tissues vulnerable to injury. A compressive force (owing to right side bending) and a rotary stress are occurring on the right side of the lumbar spine. This position also exerts a tensile force and rotary stress to the tissues on the left side of the lumbar spine.

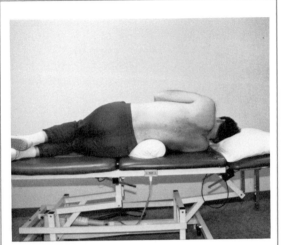

Figure 6–18. Patient is positioned right side lying over a pillow or bolster to create a stretching or lengthening force to the left lumbosacral region.

This may or may not be a nondestructive position, based on the results of the assessment. If, during the gross movement portion of the standing examination, the patient experiences his familiar pain on the left side reproduced by backward bending and side bending to the right, then this treatment position would potentially aggravate the condition. The clinician may want to enter into this potentially painful and vulnerable range, but he needs to be cautious as to the intensity of the contraction or stretch. He needs to continually assess the matches between the evaluation and the treatment process in the management of mechanical low back pain.

The point of this discussion is not to emphasize position, but rather the functional anatomy and mechanics surrounding the procedure. To explain the myriad of techniques that can be used in this phase is not within the scope of this text. The goal of the text is to assist the reader in the analysis of any technique.

One of the most common clinical challenges is to stretch the hip joint capsule and anterior thigh musculature without compromising the position of the lumbar spine. This is especially true with those patients who have a reproduction of familiar pain with the backward bend-

ing portion of the standing examination. If the clinician finds tightness of the hip when it is placed in the Faber position (Figure 4 position; see Chapter 5), or a tightness in hyperextension and internal rotation on the side of lumbopelvic pain, then stretching techniques for the tight hip are indicated. Note how tight anterior hip structures have the potential to cause anterior torsional forces of the ilium on the sacrum and extension forces on the lumbar spine when the person is in a standing posture. If the clinician stretches the anterior hip structures and at the same time creates an extension force to the lumbar spine, the healing process cannot progress. The lumbar tissue in this example remains injured, only now it is iatrogenic in nature.

The tight hip capsule and anterior hip musculature must be elongated. If they remain shortened, then the likelihood of diminishing the extension forces on the lumbar spine decreases. Therefore, the clinician is challenged with devising a stretching prescription that focuses the stretching force on the appropriate hip tissues, but renders the lumbar spine invulnerable. Figure 6–19 shows methods of stretching the hip for this clinical example.

Lastly, the patient must be continually counseled as to the movement patterns or static postures that have the potential to replicate the offending forces; or conversely, they must commit to periods of rest in optimal postures. For example, the extended posture from a prone or standing position removes the tensile force on all tissues posterior to the axis of rotation for flexion of the lumbar spine. If these patients have a reproduction of the familiar pain during the forward bending portion of the standing examination, then this posture may be effective in optimizing the healing process. With the preponderance of bending and lifting injuries, pain with forward bending or with forward bending and side bending occurs frequently, and the maintenance of the lordotic curve minimizes the tensile forces on the posterior tissues and improves the healing potential.

Potential sacroiliac lesions should be viewed in the same manner. For example, a one-legged standing posture has the potential to increase the rotary and upward shear force of the ilium

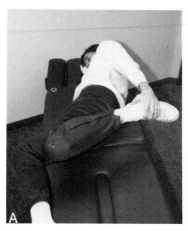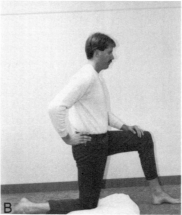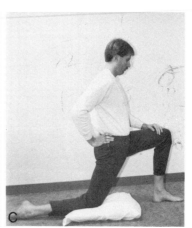

Figure 6–19.   *A,* Side lying stretching position for the anterior thigh musculature, hip flexors, and anterior hip joint capsule. The patient should be instructed as to the position of his pelvis as the force of the stretch reaches it from below. The patient should contract his abdominal wall to check the anterior rotary force that is imparted to it as the stretching force reaches the pelvis. This anterior checking of the pelvis by the abdominal wall minimizes the extension and anterior shear to the lumbar spine. It is this motion to the lumbar spine that must be protected to decreases the chances for injury during the stretch. *B,* Another example of anterior thigh, hip flexor, and anterior hip capsule stretch in a kneeling position. The patient kneels on a pillow with the leg that is to be stretched. *C,* The patient then moves forward at the hip joint. The right hand is placed on the right posterior pelvis so that an anterior and inferior force can be directed to the pelvis. This augments the stretch. The patient is instructed as to the position of his spine in relation to his pelvis. The spine should be kept in a neutral position to minimize the anterior shear and extension force to the lumbar spine.

on the sacrum owing to the convergence of forces as they reach this area (Fig. 6–20). If the evaluation has determined that these same forces reproduce this pain, then it is important for the patient to realize that it is not only one-legged standing that has the potential to be a painful stimulus, but also any posterior rotary or upward shear force of the ilium on the sacrum. It is important for the clinician and the patient to evaluate the patient's daily activities and recognize when these destructive forces might occur. Examples of potential stresses to the sacroiliac joint include squatting, end-range trunk flexion, stair-climbing, and sexual positions that place the femur in the end-range flexed, abducted, and externally rotated position.[20]

The use of a spinal orthosis can be continued during phase two. The patient must recognize

that the orthosis cannot offer complete immobility of the region. He must be cognizant of his activities, to avoid reinjury. One of the goals of the rehabilitation program is to discontinue use of the orthosis.

Phase Three

Phase three emphasizes exercise and restoration of function, and should be used in conjunction with the techniques of the second phase whenever possible.

The use of activity and exercise to manage low back problems is certainly not a new thought. Yet, until recently, this technqiue has not been the first choice for pain management, and in fact appeared to fall out of favor. This is because the main mode of treatment, perhaps

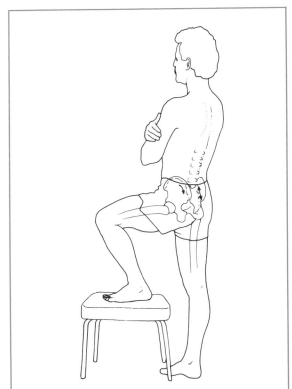

Figure 6–20. Example of the forces that reach the lumbosacral region while standing on one leg. This increases the posterior rotary moment of the ilium in an upward shear force of the ilium on the sacrum as the forces converge in this region.

tion. There is no evidence that activity is harmful, and it does not necessarily aggravate the pain. Quite to the contrary, it has been suggested that people with a high level of fitness have fewer episodes of low back pain, and if they do have an episode, they recover from it quicker.[2,3,14] In further support of using activity as a mainstay of treatment, it is clear that inactivity and prolonged rest lead to depression and distress, whereas regular activity tends to improve this condition.

With an increased understanding of the biomechanics and functional anatomy of the trunk, it is possible to avoid specific activities that are known to increase the load or excessive forces on the spine.[25] This information, plus that gained in the assessment that further identifies the increased response of the spine to specifically directed forces, allows for controlled activity and exercise to be started very early.

Why did exercise fall into disfavor? There are probably a number of reasons. One reason is that exercises tended to be given as a "program." A standardized set of exercises, such as "flexion exercises" or "extension exercises," was prescribed for patients, and then the efficacy of the exercises was compared with other therapeutic interventions, such as modalities, manipulation, and analgesics. This method has three serious flaws that need to be carefully examined.

First, the prescription of a standardized set of exercises is based on the assumption that each patient has the exact same problem. This means that the clinician's evaluation of each patient has determined that every patient requires lengthening of tissues on the posterior aspect of the trunk and strengthening of the abdominal wall to warrant a "flexion" package. The "extension" package assumes that the patient requires lengthening of tissues on the anterior side of the axis of flexion-extension motion and perhaps strengthening of the posterior tissues. Many times none of these deficiencies are even measured on the patient, but rather the exercise program is given to the patient for the sake of convenience and because of the clinician's bias toward that particular school of thought. A standardized set of exercises for low back pain is just as absurd as a standardized set

driven by the political, legal, and socioeconomic climate, was one of protracted rest, and the emphasis was on treating this problem as a disability. Activity was viewed as harmful and as something that would exacerbate the problem.

In reality, low back pain is typically benign and self-limiting. Nevertheless, the number of surgical and non-surgical treatment approaches for this problem greatly exceeds the number of such approaches for any other musculoskeletal lesion. Low back disorders have been elevated to disabilities. Waddell[25] astutely pointed out that some patients with simple low back pain are treated as if they were more seriously ill than patients with myocardial infarction, who routinely receive early ambula-

of exercises for shoulder pain or standardized surgery for all knee pain.

Second, to compare exercise with any other therapeutic intervention disregards advances made in the basic science of tissue-healing and fails to take into account the ultimate goals of a rehabilitation process, which is to restore function. The important point is that any therapeutic intervention must be appropriate for the particular stage of healing and the goal of treatment. A decrease in pain and return to function may exist simultaneously, but they cannot be equated for comparison purposes. The outcome to be measured *and* compared can be either decreased pain or increased function. Therefore, to compare the efficacy of medication or various pain-modulating techniques with the efficacy of exercise for the treatment of low back disorders is essentially meaningless. The desired outcome from each of these interventions is unique, and depends on the phase of the rehabilitation process.

Lastly, we have not advanced the technique of exercise for the trunk to the same level as that for other areas of the body. The exercise modes, from the simple curl up to the use of complex machinery, treat the muscular system as an entity divorced from the nervous system, with little regard for actual trunk muscle function and the synergistic relations between the musculature of the extremities and the trunk in order to perform a task. There also is little regard for the importance of proprioceptive and kinesthetic awareness of spine movement or positioning. Although it may be appropriate to start with these gross, nonspecific movement patterns, the clinician needs ultimately to consider both the dynamic and the stabilization requirements of the neuromuscular system of the spine for exercise to be effective.

This is comparable to our current level of understanding in dealing with hand, shoulder, or knee rehabilitation. At some point function that requires proprioceptive and kinesthetic awareness and that relies on afferent and efferent information to and from the central nervous system must be introduced. The clinician has learned that a 100 per cent comparison of right and left quadriceps strength on an isokinetic test does not result in increased jumping ability, nor does a 100 per cent comparison of

right and left grip strength translate into the ability to quickly unfasten buttons or manipulate the environment with dexterity. Instead, the ultimate goals from rehabilitation of the knee and hand include some degree of proprioceptive training. In addition, the clinician has recognized the importance of both the specificity of exercise and the restoration of function appropriate for the demands that will ultimately be placed on the injured area in each case. The same consideration should be given to the trunk.

Training of the neuromusculoskeletal system is the desired outcome of the exercise program. Training prepares the body to adapt to stressful situations.[5,22] For many low back patients the learning of spinal movement through invulnerable ranges itself is considered training. For others exercises to develop strength, endurance, and coordination are also considered training. A training program affects not only the muscle tissue, but also the nervous system.[8] The increase in stiffness of the muscle as a result of training enhances the muscle tissue's ability to attenuate forces. Likewise, the increase in strength as a result of training is partly due to the ability of the central nervous system to effectively recruit motor units and effectively balance motor unit activation of both the agonists and the antagonists. This is essential for purposeful, controlled movement.

Therefore, the term *training* should not be limited in definition, but include all approaches used to encourage and improve function. Techniques to improve movement awareness include proprioceptive neuromuscular facilitation, sensory integration, Feldenkrais, and Tai-Chi, as well as various resistance exercises. These are all forms of training because of their neuromotoric, hypertrophic, and mechanical influences.

During this phase supports are discontinued except when the patient is involved in strenuous physical activity, especially those activities that replicate the mechanism of injury. Training of the muscular system with resistance exercises can begin with recognition of two guidelines:

1.   Initial use of a protected or invulnerable range as determined by the assessment (see Figs. 6–4 and 6–5)

2. A progression of difficulty from non-weight-bearing positions to weight-bearing positions that require complex motor patterns

What is a protected range? The patient must learn to recognize the difference between the vulnerable and the invulnerable position of his lumbopelvic tissues. This position is unique to the individual, and depends on his history. For example, if extension of the lumbar spine reproduces the painful stimulus, and this pain increases with overpressure, then any exercise that subjects the lumbopelvic region to increased extension and compression force makes this area vulnerable to reinjury.

This can be compared with the patient whose pain pattern is reproduced with flexion-type movements of the lumbar spine. For this person it is preferable to begin a training program with exercises that have a minimal chance of introducing a flexion force. A flexion force can reach the lumbar spine from the ground up or the trunk down. A position of spinal extension or a normal lumbar lordosis is desired in this example. A curl up, which allows trunk flexion, is an inappropriate exercise for this patient.

Granted that these two examples are straightforward and simplistic, but they are chosen to emphasize the relation between the assessment and the exercise prescription. The same thought processes need to occur with torsional, compressive, shear, and multiplane forces. In both of the examples above, the goal is to initiate resistance exercises and begin the important aspect of training by teaching the patient to maintain an invulnerable position of his spine.

Starting a program in this manner is important because it is the first attempt to train the trunk muscles as *stabilizers*, rather than *prime movers*. This type of activity might best be termed proprioceptive and kinesthetic training of the trunk, since the muscles are asked to control spinal position based on afferent neurologic input, which increases awareness of spinal positions.

The second guideline refers to the progression of exercises, and takes advantage of non-

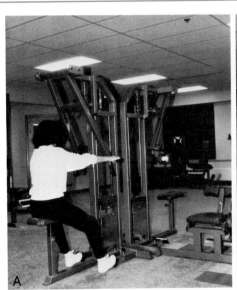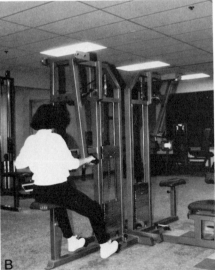

Figure 6–21. Seated maximum-protection pulling-type exercises. *A*, Patient is stabilized in the front with a pad and the feet are fixed on foot plates. The pelvis is then fixed, and *B*, the patient pulls back.

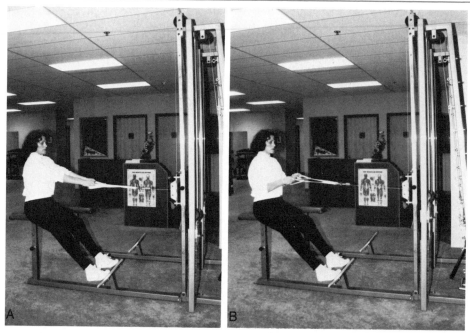

Figure 6–22.   Seated cable row with seat fixed in a high position to minimize the flexion moment in the spine. *A*, The patient maintains spinal position and then *B*, pulls back without motion in her spine.

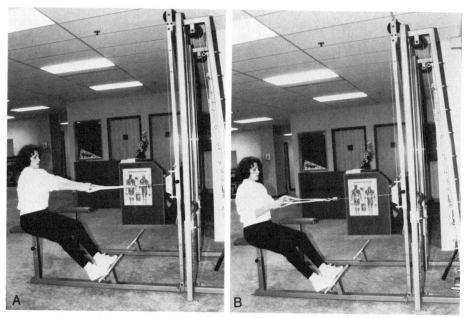

Figure 6–23.   Seated cable row, low seating position. *A, B,* This position decreases the extension moment and increases the flexion moment in the spine. The seat height can be placed at any position to maintain the weight-bearing process in a nondestructive manner.

weight-bearing positions from which the patient can begin resistance exercises while having an easier time controlling spinal position. Single-plane exercises are chosen initially because they are easier for the patient to accomplish. This impacts greatly on the degree of difficulty of the exercise. As soon as the trunk assumes a weight-bearing function and must also attenuate trunk and ground forces, the degree of difficulty in moving through or maintaining an invulnerable spinal position dramatically increases. Figures 6–21 through 6–31

show various pulling exercises from the supine, sitting, and standing positions. The reader should recognize the increased demands on the neuromusculoskeletal system with the change of positions and the progression from single-plane to multiplane activities.

Failure to adhere to these two guidelines is one of the major pitfalls in the attempt to move a patient form the confines of the clinical setting to the community exercise facility. The patient is only told to continue exercise, but he does not understand the vulnerable spinal mo-

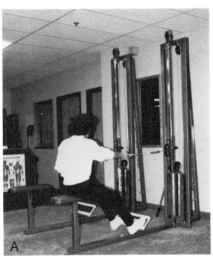 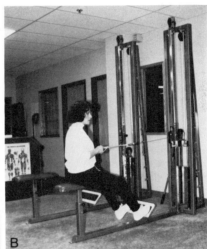

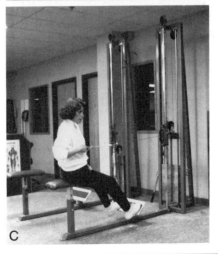

Figure 6–24. Seated cable row, cross rowing. *A*, Patient is placed in a neutral position and encouraged to maintain the position of her pelvis. *B*, She is then asked to pull with her right arm back and *C*, around to improve the strength of her scapular retractors and rotators. This position increases the rotary moment in the spine as compared to Figure 6–23.

tions or positions. He is unable to maintain the invulnerable positions while using the multitude of exercise machines that necessitate supine, prone, sitting, or standing positions.

The principles guiding this type of proprioceptive and kinesthetic strength training should also be followed for any exercise equipment for the lower or upper extremities, free weights, ergometers, treadmills, and all forms of low- and high-impact aerobic dance. Exercise monitoring for these patients must be done by health care professionals who have a comprehensive knowledge of functional anatomy of the trunk and assessment skills, rather than by untrained instructors.

In the standing position multiplane movement patterns with resistance present the greatest degree of difficulty. This is due to the necessity of recruiting and contracting the trunk and the upper- and lower-extremity muscle groups in a smooth, coordinated manner so that the weight-bearing line remains controlled as it traverses the lumbopelvic tissues. The emphasis shifts to the quality of the motion rather than the quantity, and underscores the importance of body awareness.

For example, an exercise with pulleys or elasticized resistance that uses a pulling motion requires a coordinated effort of the shoulder extensors, scapula retractors, and spine

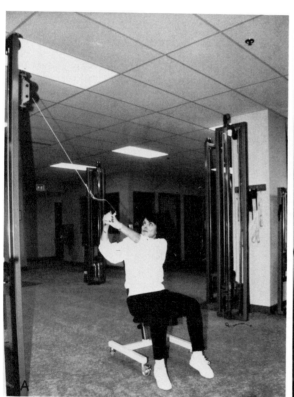
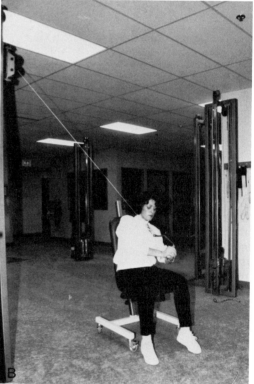

Figure 6–25. Seated cross pull down with an upper pulley position. A, Patient is seated in a high-back chair to increase the stability of the spine. B, She is then asked to pull down and across with emphasis on pulling the right inferior aspect of the rib cage toward the left anterior superior iliac spine. This is an excellent exercise for the anterior trunk, and the posterior aspect of the trunk is stabilized with the seat.

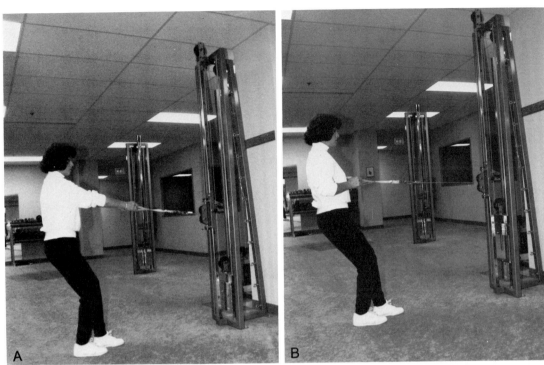

Figure 6–26. Standing cable pulls with the pulley in the mid position. *A,* Patient is asked to stand with one foot in front of the other to neutralize her base of support and decrease the anterior shear on her spine. *B,* Then she pulls back, not allowing any motion of the trunk.

extensors at the very minimum. If we super-impose on this activity the idea of maintaining an invulnerable position of the lumbopelvic re-gion, we add significant involvement of the muscles that control the pelvis and lumbar spine, such as the deep erector spinae, multif-idus, abdominals, hip extensors, abductors, and adductors. This activity occurs by virtue of their attachments to the lumbar spine, pelvis, and femurs.

Remember, however, that to make gains in muscle strength or endurance, the point of mo-mentary failure must be approached in order to provide the stimulus for the necessary bio-chemical and anatomic changes in the mus-cle.[8,21] The muscle must be given the opportu-nity to respond to these new stresses. In the example above, the problem may not be the shoulder extensors that fail as a number of the

pulling repetitions are performed, but rather an inability to stabilize or move the trunk properly, or perhaps failure of the scapula re-tractors. Figure 6–32 shows a pulling exercise with free weights from a kneeling position in which the pulling action by the shoulder ex-tensors does not fail, but rather the inability of the trunk muscles to stabilize the trunk against excessive rotary forces.

The clinician must analyze the complete movement pattern with an eye toward all of the functioning muscle groups for the exercise. The point of failure for the activity is when any one of the linked components performing this activity no longer moves correctly or safely. Substitution, or vulnerable movement patterns occur as a result of this failure. Many times this failure occurs in the trunk, resulting in exces-sive rotary, flexion, or extension motions as the

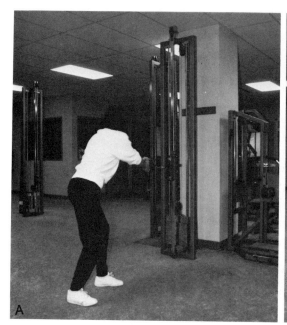

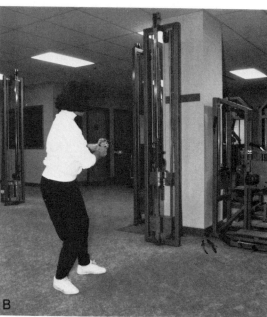

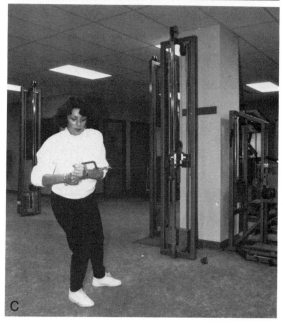

Figure 6–27.   Standing cross pulls with pulley in the mid position. *A*, Patient is placed in a comfortable position in a forward bent rotation left. *B*, The motion is pull cross the body to the opposite position and then *C*, a slow, controlled return to the starting position.

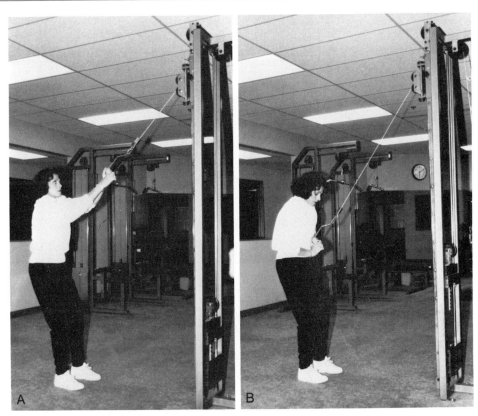

Figure 6–28.   Standing pull down with the pulley in the up position. *A*, Patient stands with her feet parallel. *B*, The motion is humeral extension and trunk flexion.

person attempts to complete the motion of the upper or lower extremity. Therefore, exercise fatigue can be defined more accurately as substitution of muscle function.

With this type of training program the concept of "3 sets of 10" is no longer appropriate because the patient may still be able to do the shoulder extension component of a pulling exercise, but the clinician immediately recognizes the inappropriate activity of the other segments. The clinician needs to alert the patient to the importance of all the components of this chain working synchronously and avoiding overload of one area. This represents the difference between the concepts of weight-

lifting and resistance training. Table 6–1 lists the differences in the terminology for weight-lifting, in which the goal is to build size and raw strength as quickly as possible, as opposed to the phase three concept of resistance training, in which the goal is neuromuscular efficiency.

For many patients with longstanding lumbopelvic problems moving the lower or upper extremities independent of the spine is difficult. The integration of the nervous and muscular systems, resulting in one neuromuscular strategy, emphasizes the importance of coordination of the trunk and extremities, and recognizes the balance between afferent and effer-

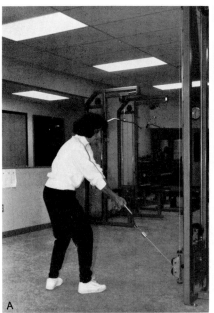

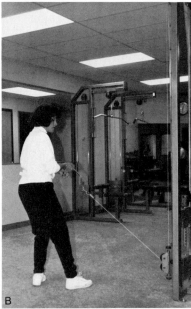

Figure 6–29. Standing cross pulls with pulley in the low position. *A–C,* This complex motion must be controlled by the large musculature of the trunk. The prime movers are the shoulders, hips, and legs. This is an excellent exercise for training the musculature of the trunk to stabilize the back so that motions can be carried out through the upper and lower extremities.

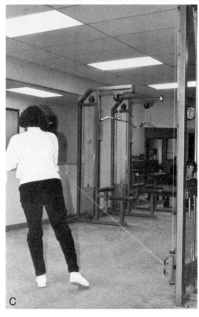

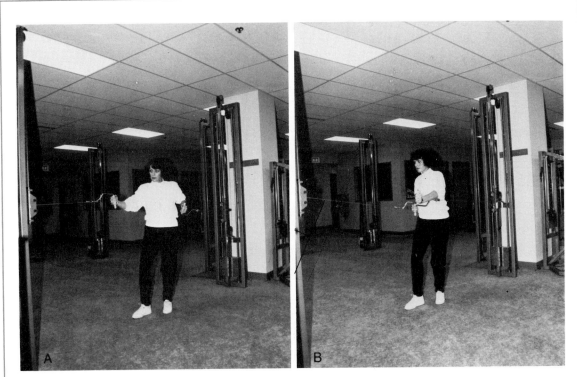

Figure 6–30. Standing cross pulls with pulleys in the neutral position. *A*, Patient stands between two vertical pulleys. She grasps a handle in each hand and then *B*, pulls with the right hand and pushes with the left. Note the activity that must take place with the internal and external obliques of the abdominal wall and the lateral guy wires of the trunk in order to carry out this motion. This is an excellent exercise to cause reciprocal contraction of the musculature of the trunk.

ent nervous system activity. Without this appropriate motor pattern, excessive torsional, shear, tensile, and compressive forces are potentially directed to the lumbopelvic tissues when the upper and lower extremities move through their range of motion. The muscles of the trunk must, therefore, be trained to dynamically stabilize this region.[19] Training in turn optimizes the ability of the muscles to accept and attenuate forces by increasing their overall stiffness.[8] It is important to relate this type of training to activities of daily living and the work environment.

Phase Four

The patient will probably be faced with limitations as a result of injury to the lumbopelvic region. They may be particular movements that need to be avoided, loads on the lumbopelvic region that might provoke symptoms, the inability to adopt certain positions, or the frequency with which the lumbopelvic area can be provoked. This phase is also an educational process. The clinician is attempting to establish the patient's movement, load, position, and frequency limitations.

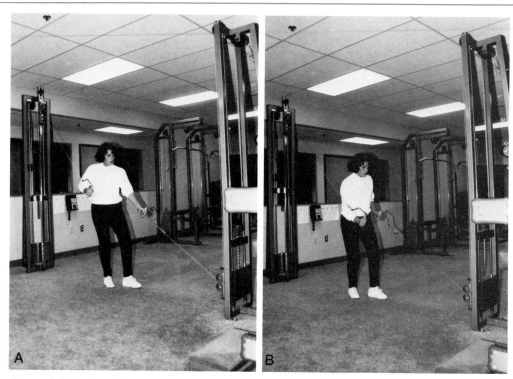

Figure 6–31. Standing cross pulls with an upper pulley and a lower pulley position. This exercise lines up the force in the direction of the oblique musculature of the trunk and, if done correctly, is probably the best abdominal wall exercise. *A*, Patient grasps each of the handles and *B*, pushes down with the right hand and at the same time pulls back with the left hand. The concentration should be in the movement of the trunk (i.e., movement of the right inferior aspect of the rib cage to the left anterior superior iliac spine). The base of support should be one foot in front of the other to enhance stability. The patient is asked to pull down, pause, and slowly return to the starting position.

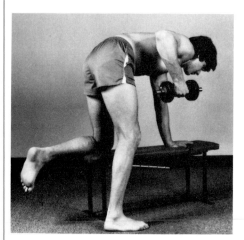

Figure 6–32. One-arm row using a bench and free weight. The patient's trunk is stabilized with the left knee on the bench and the right foot on the floor. The free weight is then pulled up and back using the latissimus, the scapular retractors, and the humeral extensors. The patient places the back in a neutral position and does not allow it to come out of position during the exercise. Once the low back begins to substitute, or change, its neutral position, the exercise should be terminated.

TABLE 6–1.   Common Terminology: Weight Lifting Versus Neuromuscular Rehabilitation Training

Weight Lifting	Resistance Training in Rehab
3 sets of 10	Sets to momentary fatigue
Isolation movements	Functional movements
Concentration	Body position awareness
Full range of motion	Nondestructive range of motion
No pain, no gain	Train, don't strain
Arms, pecs, delts	Postural muscles
Cutting up	Tissue remodeling
Maximal loading	Submaximal loading
Hypertrophy	Increasing tone/decreasing stiffness
Speed/power	Movement efficiency
Reps to failure	Reps to substitution
Athletic competition	Active lifestyle

There are many names for the various efforts to optimize the patient's physical condition and return him to his preinjured level of activity by teaching him his functional limits. From the scientific perspective, the common link between many of the "back school" and "work-hardening" programs is that they teach proprioceptive awareness of spinal motion, they attempt to increase the participant's fitness level, and they teach the patient what his limitations are. The clinician should not be confused by the different titles given to these programs, but should judge their value on their potential to achieve neuromuscular and behavior modification improvements. The value of any program is its success in teaching the patient how to manage his disability.

SUMMARY

The purpose of this chapter is to develop a logical progression of treatment formulated on the physiologic basis of tissue-healing and the goal of restoring function. There are many ways to achieve the desired result in each phase. Many times the choice of technique is influenced by the availability of the equipment or the skill of the clinician. Whichever technique is chosen, the ultimate goal of the rehabilitation process should not be lost: the resto-

ration of function by means of early activity. In the end it will be the patient who must necessarily manage his own problem.

The treatment goal in all cases is to assist the patient in maximizing the potential for functional healing and enhancing his ability to attenuate stresses in the lumbopelvic region. This goal is accomplished by optimizing the patient's ability to control the forces of gravity and movement by means of balancing anatomic structure and improving neuromuscular efficiency. This treatment protocol takes time and patience, but without a goal-oriented, phased rehabilitation process that encourages restoration of function, the clinician has no hope of producing lasting results in the treatment of lumbopelvic disorders.

REFERENCES

1. Berquist-Ullman M, Larsson U: Acute lowback pain in industry. Acta Orthop Scand (Suppl) 170:1, 1977.
2. Biering-Soresen P: Physical measurements as risk indicators for lowback trouble over a one year period. Spine 9:106, 1984.
3. Cady L, Bischoff D, O'Connel E: Strength and fitness and subsequent back injuries in firefighters. J Occup Med 21:269, 1979.
4. Cyriax J: Textbook of Orthopedic Medicine, vol 1. London, Bailliere-Tindall, 1978.
5. Fleck SJ, Falkel JE: Value of resistance training for the reduction of sports injuries. Sports Med 3:61, 1986.
6. Forrest I: Current concepts in soft connective tissue wound healing. Br J Surg 70:133, 1983.
7. Kellett J: Acute soft tissue injuries—a review of the literature. Med Sci Sports Exerc 18:489, 1986.
8. Komi PV: Training of muscle strength and power: Interaction of neuromotoric, hypertrophic and mechanical factors. Int J Sports Med 7(Suppl):10, 1986.
9. Mayer TG, Gatchel RJ: Functional Restoration for Spinal Disorders: The Sports Medicine Approach. Philadelphia, Lea & Febiger, 1988, p 36.
10. Mayer TG, Kishino N, Keeley J, et al: Using physical measurements to assess lowback pain. J Musc Med 2:44, 1985.
11. McMaster PE: Tendon and muscle ruptures. J Bone Joint Surg 15:705, 1933.
12. Mixter WJ, Barr JS: Rupture of the intervertebral disc with involvement of the spinal canal. N Engl J Med 211:210, 1934.
13. Mooney V: Where is the pain coming from? Presidential address, International Society for the Study of the Lumbar Spine. Spine 12:754, 1987.
14. Nachemson A: Work for all, for those with lowback pain as well. Clin Orthop 179:77, 1983.
15. Nikolaou PK, Macdonald BL, Glisson RR, et al: Bio-

mechanical and histological evaluation of muscle after controlled strain injury. Am J Sports Med 15:9, 1987.

16. Noyes FR, DeLucas JL, Torvik PJ: Biomechanics of anterior cruciate ligament failure: An analysis of strain-rate sensitivity and mechanisms of failure in primates. J Bone Joint Surg [AM] 56A:236, 1974.

17. Noyes FR, Grood ES, Butler DL, et al: Clinical laxity tests and functional stability of the knee: Biomechanical concepts. Clin Orthop 146:84, 1980.

18. Panjabi MM, Krag MH, Chung TQ: Effects of disc injury on mechanical behavior of the human spine. Spine 9:707, 1984.

19. Porterfield JA: Dynamic stabilization of the trunk. J Orthop Sports Phys Ther 6:271, 1985.

20. Porterfield JA, DeRosa CP: The sacroiliac joint. In Gould JA (ed): Orthopedic and Sports Physical Therapy, 2nd edition. St. Louis, CV Mosby, 1990, p 553.

21. Sale DG, MacDougall JD, Upton ARM, McComas AJ: Effect of strength training upon motoneuron excitability in man. Med Sci Sports Exerc 15:57, 1983.

22. Stone MH: Implications for connective tissue and bone alterations resulting from resistance exercise training. Med Sci Sports Exerc 20(Suppl):S162, 1988.

23. Troup J: Driver's back pain and its prevention: A review of the postural, vibratory and muscular factors, together with the problem of transmitted road shock. Appl Ergonom 9:207, 1978.

24. van der Muelen JCH: Present state of knowledge on processes of healing in collagen structures. Int J Sports Med 3:4, 1982.

25. Waddell G: A new clinical model for the treatment of lowback pain. Spine 12:632, 1987.

26. Wiesel SW, Tsourmas N, Feffer HL, et al: A study of computer assisted tomography: The incidence of positive CAT scans in an asymptomatic group of patients. Spine 9:549, 1984.

27. Wyke B: Neurological aspects of low back pain. In Jayson M (ed): The Lumbar Spine and Back Pain. New York, Grune & Stratton, p 189, 1976.

28. Zarins B: Soft tissue injury and repair—biomechanical aspects. Int J Sports Med 3:9, 1982.

INDEX

ARAPAHOE COMMUNITY COLLEGE

3 1717 00⬛⬛⬛⬛56

⬛⬛⬛⬛⬛ B217 P67 1991
Porterfield, James A.
Mechanical low back pain

DAT